EMBODY WHOLENESS

Guided Shamanic Techniques for
Transforming Trauma into Well-Being

2nd Edition

JUDITH HOAGLUND

ISBN 979-8-9935767-0-1 (print)
ISBN 979-8-9935767-1-8 (ebook)
ISBN 979-8-9935767-2-5 (audiobook)

Second Edition
Inner Wholeness Press
Santa Rosa, California
Printed in the United States of America.

Cover design by Gordon D. Beebe

Contents

Forward

READING JUDITH HOAGLUND'S PRECIOUS AND selfless book, <u>Embody Wholeness</u>, I can't avoid contrasting it with the numerous advertisements of self-appointed shamans who, for a fee, offer vision quests, sweats, naming ceremonies or other plundered esoterica from America's indigenous people. I would never want you to confuse Judith Hoaglund with that ilk. Judith is a straightforward, compassionate and powerful healer and teacher.

She has spent decades of study under elders, teachers and masters in Mexico, Peru and the U.S., but what will amaze you in her book is the breadth of her insight, and her generosity in offering gifts which you can apply in your own journey of healing.

Whether it is an illness for which Western medicine has no answers, a fragmented sense of self, "archived energies," or the deep and lasting traumas of infancy, childhood, family and ancestors, her ability to transform and heal, using her complement of shamanic techniques in explorations of self, entities, and afflictions, is remarkable and life-altering. She is made of and behaves with integrity. As one who can speak from personal experience, she can lead you to and through genuine healing.

PETER COYOTE, AUTHOR, ZEN BUDDHIST PRIEST AND TEACHER

Second Edition Preface

IN THIS NEW EDITION, I have made a few changes to reflect how I am currently using these modalities in my healing practice, and to further clarify some of the methods that have already been presented. Two new chapters have been added that will give practitioners more information, inspiration and scope of practice for working with their clients. Most of the references to hypnosis have been removed or altered. The feedback I received from both clients and readers indicated that my use of those terms contributed to confusion or created unnecessary barriers to the practice of the healing modalities without adding any significant benefit.

Over many years of reading books on a variety of approaches to healing and the various methodologies employed, it has been the case studies in those books that have impressed me the most. For me personally, detailed case studies have been extremely helpful, both for their educational value and also as a springboard for kindling new ideas, approaches, ways of understanding issues and expanded possibilities for the work I do. In that light, I have added more case studies as food for thought.

I continue to be amazed at the profound depth of healing that is facilitated by the spirit guides who are ever ready to assist people in need. It has also been extremely gratifying to receive numerous reports from readers who are now successfully using these shamanic techniques to provide effective and lasting healing to their own clients.

Practitioners frequently comment to me that, at first, they were skeptical of the potency and practicality of the modalities in this book, saying that they seemed too simple to be truly effective. Once they actually used these techniques and witnessed first-hand their capacity to clear and heal myriad client complaints, they couldn't wait to share their successes with me.

I sincerely encourage anyone interested in health and well-being to put the information shared in this book into practice. I am confident that you will find it to be of value to you, both personally and in your practice of energy healing.

JUDITH HOAGLUND, MS
NORTHERN CALIFORNIA
SEPTEMBER 27, 2025

Preface

IF I HAD KNOWN ABOUT energy healing as a child, I likely would have picked that topic to write about in my fourth-grade essay on "What I want to be when I grow up." My journey toward the spiritual aspects of energy healing actually did start in childhood, as, at age seven, I was consumed with the question "Who am I?"—and I have been asking it ever since. I have always known that there is considerably more happening in our midst than what our five senses tell us, but I could find no one interested in exploring nonphysical realms, communicating with plants, with ancient ancestors or extraterrestrials. My searching was inexorably crushed by the consensual reality of my family and friends. I found no support, no guidance, nor even language for the non-ordinary experiences I had as a child. Nor did I encounter what I sought in the myriad religions, philosophies or sciences I studied, and I began to forget about seeking. The only place, then and now, where I consistently feel whole, seen and supported is when I am in nature—the wilder and more remote, the better.

At age 27, I had a profound mystical experience that launched me into a renewed search for spiritual dimensions. At that time, I identified as an atheist and had chosen biological science as the main focus of my life and studies. I believed in the Universe and everything in it yet saw it all through the lens of the classic, mechanistic and even Darwinian systems that my science education had assured me it was. Some part of me still knew that there was more to existence than three-dimensional reality, but I had deeply buried those feelings to align myself with accepted cultural beliefs. This confining myopic ideology was utterly shattered by my direct experience of the Divine. I will share a brief description of my experience to try to convey the transformative nature of this encounter.

I was lying in bed late one afternoon with intense emotional angst, feeling as if my life was rapidly collapsing around me. I suddenly found myself in an experiential vision where I was falling and falling, ever deeper, into an abyss of despair. This abyss was utterly black—I could see nothing. It was inconceivably deep and absolutely terrifying. As I felt myself endlessly falling, I had only one thought: I knew for sure if I hit the bottom of that pit, I would be extinguished as a being. Not only would I cease to exist, but I would also never have existed and would never again exist as any form of consciousness.

The prospect of this rapidly-approaching total annihilation was unnerving. The abyss was an absolute void. There was nothing: nothing I could do, no way out, no options; nothing but falling, deeper and deeper. In the illogic of my dread, I felt that there simply could not be nothing—there had to be something, and, if there was anything at all, it would have to be God. The fact that I did not believe in God was thoroughly irrelevant, and so I prayed with the entirety of my being, "Oh, God! Please save me!"

Instantly, two enormous, glowing, golden "hands of God" caught me and stopped my fall. My relief at being miraculously saved was dwarfed by the immense love that flooded into me. I received what I would now call a download of insight, information and knowledge in that moment. My entire life, identity and sense of myself forever changed, and I was awash in gnosis beyond retention. I understood that all of my education, cultural conditioning, beliefs, everything that I thought I knew—and even my very self—were a mere drop in the ocean of All That Is. As if a cosmic reset button had been pushed, I started over and received a new life. In the months that followed, even though the ineffable experience faded, I again became consumed with the search to understand what lies outside Western culture's accepted understanding of reality. I remembered my childhood quest for the Great Mystery of Being and put it back in the center of my life.

My subsequent exploration led me to studies of the world's mystical religious traditions. Here, at least, people understood and experienced transcendent states of consciousness and the great unknown. I spent decades immersed in Sufism, becoming a disciple of this form of alchemical mysticism, as it reshaped my life. I focused intensely on the wisdom teachings of healing and transformation of consciousness. Eventually, and as I look back at that now, it appears that when I reached the limit of what I could digest and absorb from this tradition, my life fell apart again. When that door closed, as the saying goes, another one opened.

I left the mystical path to plumb the depths of earth-based traditions, entering into the exploration of shamanic realms and sacred plant medicines, again becoming a disciple of these arts and lineage teachings. Wending my way through another decades-long sojourn, I fortuitously received wisdom and guidance from many elders, ancestors, teachers and spirit allies in the U.S., Mexico and Peru. As I gained experience and knowledge in these realms, I created a private healing practice to assist others in the journey of healing and awakening, and this became a source of deep nourishment.

As my search continued, I encountered the Pachakuti Mesa Tradition®, a cross-cultural shamanic path, where I committed to an in-depth apprenticeship into Peruvian healing and earth-honoring traditions. For many years, I devoted myself entirely to the ancient wisdom, practices and cosmology of the Andes, expanding my healing capacity, experience and intuition in the process. Eventually, I became a sanctioned teacher of this mesa lineage and taught immersive apprenticeships for another decade.

My healing service deepened, and I felt pulled into surrendering to my purpose, vision, and what I had come here to create during this lifetime. Throughout my forty-year-plus experiential journey, I had been conducting spiritual healing work of various types on everyone who came to me for help. From focused prayer and remote healing for individuals, groups and the collective, my service evolved over the years into what you will read about in this book—a spiritual, in-person and hands-on energy healing practice. I amassed many techniques, modalities, approaches, and an augmented understanding of ever-expanding healing potential through direct experience and enthusiastic reading. Over the years, I traveled widely, visiting 20 countries and living for a year or more in three of them. This blessing exposed me to many cultures. The experience of living in other cultures was priceless, and as anyone who has done so knows, it changed me in ways I never dreamed possible.

Over the years of immersion, apprenticing, study and initiations, I added Reiki, breathwork, hypnotherapy, meditation, trance dance, energy healing, sacred plant wisdom and numerous shamanic techniques to my medicine bag. The healing modalities presented here gradually emerged in an organic, alchemical process. As I applied these different therapies to my clients' eclectic health challenges, I began to witness remarkable results—people I worked with transformed before my eyes. My guides continually encouraged me to expand my healing work and gave me incredible, intuitive insights as I worked with clients.

As a life philosophy, I have shared my knowledge with anyone genuinely interested in accessing it. Thus, throughout the years of energy healing practice, I taught my clients to use the techniques I was using on them during their sessions. I observed that nearly everyone could remember and use the processes on themselves and even on others. As I grew older, I understood the importance of passing on my experience, tools and cosmology to more people. In other words, I wanted to integrate all that I had gleaned and offer it back to Source in a form that promoted optimum healing for everyone who encountered it.

I received strong guidance to begin teaching groups, and this became the manner in which I shared my knowledge with others who would, in turn, use it and share it more widely. This teaching took the form of weekend experiential workshops, which began with small groups of students who shared my enthusiasm for shamanic healing. My students loved and appreciated the workshops and gave enthusiastic feedback that prompted me to teach more.

During each workshop, profound participant healing stories emerged, and as the groups shared their insights, our collective experience broadened exponentially. I began receiving significant reports from former students recounting stories of the surprising therapeutic results they were having with their clients. The realization that these energy healing techniques are teachable, reproducible and powerfully effective began to weigh heavily on me. I felt a growing responsibility to do more.

Numerous clients and friends had told me, over the years, that I should write a book or that they "saw" me writing a book. I did not doubt that I would eventually write one, but the problem was that I could not yet "see" this book. I had amassed many healing stories but didn't know how or where to begin to tell them. I knew that a book could reach large numbers of people, but somehow that was not enough. Years went by, and I figured if I was meant to write a book, Spirit would give me some pointers.

On May 1, 2020, after sheltering in place for most of March and all of April due to the COVID-19 pandemic, I awoke to "my book." I could suddenly see it in its entirety, and it was all so clear, easy and straightforward. Why had it been so hard for me to see it earlier? The answer I received by asking this question was "Divine timing." I got up, sat at the computer, and within an hour had an entire outline of my book typed up, along with other notes to myself about resources, allies and potential publishers. As I sat there, information, stories, ideas and long-forgotten memories came pouring out. I was in the zone.

Thus, I can say I am grateful to COVID-19 for giving me the time I needed to gestate and write this book. With the shelter-in-place mandate, all my workshops were canceled or indefinitely put on hold, perhaps never again to happen in person. I had plenty of free time; no clients were coming to me, nor could I make any appointments in our sequestered world. I felt incredibly blessed to have no personal worries about my health or well-being and proceeded with my plan for an extended writer's retreat. I realized the pandemic presented a golden opportunity for me to become more creative and to accomplish this significant goal.

For whom is this book written? Anyone interested in the role of energy, consciousness and spiritual development, as it applies to healing, will likely enjoy this book. It is for healers of any kind: energy healing practitioners, shamanic practitioners, therapists, counselors, hypnotherapists, social workers, psychologists, acupuncturists, bodyworkers or anyone curious about shamanic and energy healing, self-healing, ancestor/transgenerational healing, or healing family and friends. The scope of this healing is indeed quantum—pulling from the field of infinite potentiality.

The modalities described in this book can be used to address myriad physical, mental, emotional and even spiritual concerns in addition to illness, and are particularly applicable to those conditions for which conventional medicine has no effectual answers. These techniques provide a drug-free method to address and resolve the core issues from which dis-ease arises instead of simply treating, sedating or masking symptoms. The processes presented evolved from heart-centered wisdom traditions and real-life practice involving many hundreds of people over several decades. The techniques are simple and straightforward, yet not simplistic—and anyone who reads this book will glean enough information to begin addressing dis-ease in themselves, as well as in others.

Dr. Gabor Maté, a well-known psychiatrist and expert in the fields of trauma and addiction, stresses that most physical, emotional and mental illness originates in coping patterns that developed to address infancy and childhood trauma. Most people I have met carry emotional baggage from these early experiences. The modalities in this book can address this archived energy. Examples of conditions impacted include a wide variety of conditions: pain syndromes, depression, anxiety, panic attacks, sexual and physical abuse, anger, addictions, compulsions, obsessions, phobias, autoimmune disorders, stress, relationship issues, inherited family trauma and more.

The healing that people experience through these therapeutic energy modalities is real, lasting and profound. Since all healing is accomplished by Spirit, the power of these techniques lies in their ability to convey an individual to this healing Source. Whether or not—and the degree to which—the healing transpires depends on variables we cannot possibly know. In many Indigenous traditions, healers understand that there are two types of illness: that which may be cured and that which may not be cured because it is a vital part of a person's life plan. Even those with so-called incurable diseases may obtain precise information about why they have such a condition, the purpose it serves in their life, and potential treatments and healing.

There is nothing exceptional about me as a healing practitioner. I am intuitive and empathic but do not consider myself unusually gifted, sensitive, clairvoyant or psychic. Special skills are not required for this type of work, as long as a person is aligned with great integrity and Source and holds the intention to be of selfless service for the highest good of all. Anyone willing to apply themselves to the processes and open to higher consciousness and spiritual guidance can learn these healing techniques. I also believe these modalities are widely applicable to more than healing, as they hold the potential to solve other problems a person might have. For example, one can receive personal coaching and advice from one's higher guides via these methods.

This is a "how-to" book. Its purpose is to teach others how to use the healing modalities presented. I explain the various processes that I use to facilitate healing with my clients and provide case studies to illustrate how they work. Appendix I contains a summary of these processes, making them easier to locate for quick reference.

In Appendix II, I present letters from students and clients with whom I have worked. I include them because they represent viewpoints from those receiving this quantum energy healing and express the impact the work has had on them. The case studies presented are my actual case studies collected over the years. I should note that some of the accounts I share have potentially disturbing content. I have removed the more graphic details yet want to forewarn energetically sensitive people.

All personal names and identifying characteristics have been changed to protect client privacy. I have also omitted the names of most of the higher guides.

We are on the brink of a phenomenal healing revolution with new, radical understanding and breakthrough technologies emerging continually. I desire to spark your imagination and fuel your inquiry into the realms of spirit-based energy healing and to wish you well as a fellow traveler through the Great Mystery of Being.

Judith Hoaglund, MS
Northern California
February 1, 2021

Chapter 1

Healing Depths

THE EARLY MORNING SUN WAS filtering through the large live oak trees to the east. Enjoying my morning cup of tea on the patio, I mused about what I would do on this bright and cheerful spring day. The jarring sound of the phone ringing inside the house abruptly brought me out of my reverie. I jumped up to get the call, scattering songbirds that were feeding in our backyard. It was from a woman named Anne. She explained that her good friend, Marcie, had studied with me several years before and recommended she call me. After a brief chat, I asked Anne to give me a general idea of the work she wanted to do. She sounded like a person who was desperate for healing, and I listened closely to her words. After asking her a few questions, I told her that I felt I could help her. We set an appointment for her to come to my home on the following Tuesday morning.

As I opened the door for Anne, I could see she was a woman who carried deep wounds. The sad expression in her eyes, combined with her quiet and somber demeanor, gave me the feeling that Anne's journey had been long and hard. She was middle-aged, with long brown hair that spilled over her shoulders. She had on a simple blouse and long flowing skirt and wore many necklaces with beads, crystals and talismans. I felt instant compassion for her and gave her a hug as I welcomed her into my healing room. I oriented her to my sacred altar, the focal point of our work and the place where she would be sitting for the session. My large altar rests on the floor and occupies a predominant portion of the small room. It contains numerous crystals, shells, candles, feathers, stones, photographs and artifacts from my travels, arranged to honor the cardinal directions. I explained a bit about the energy healing work and asked if she had any questions. Anne said she liked the rainbow colors of my altar and all the masks that hang on the wall next to it. She felt comfortable, relaxed and held by my healing room, so I invited her to join me in opening sacred space for our session together.

As we grounded ourselves, activated the altar and called in our higher guides to support our work, I observed that Anne was an energetically sensitive person. She told me that she could feel the power of my altar and that it was like sitting in front of a small bonfire, filling her with warmth and safety. I encouraged her to elaborate on her life issues and the healing she had accomplished so far. She explained that she had a history of trauma that encompassed her entire life, beginning in utero. Her mother did not want to be pregnant and tried to abort Anne and her twin sister with a combination of knitting needles and drugs. This drastic approach resulted in the death of the twin, which, Anne remarked, she still remembered. She was sure that even now she carried deep trauma from that time which she had never been able to resolve, describing it as a dull ache in her soul.

Anne continued, saying she was aware of what she termed "toxic damage" to her brain from her life experiences, which caused unclear thinking and brain fog. She also confided that she was in constant fear, as if something evil was always lurking just out of sight or around a corner. Anne's many years of therapy had been life- and sanity-saving, yet she sensed there was more to do that therapy just couldn't reach. She had heard from her friend Marcie that the work I did reached these deeper levels buried in the psyche.

I asked Anne if she knew the source of her intractable fear. Here the story dramatically deepened, and she explained that, from infancy to about three years old, she had been ritually tortured by the members of a dark cult. She gave me many details of the horrors she had survived. It was a shock to hear her full story, even though this was not the first time I had encountered and worked with this type of trauma. She explained that her father had been a member of this sinister group, even offering his daughter for their rituals. In it, members tapped into the energies of sex and death, apparently more for self-gratification than for personal power or black magic.

For years, Anne was subjected to extreme and painful abuse, which finally ended with her father's premature death. Even now, she retained some visceral memories of these early events, which trailed behind her like a heavy chain. Through the years of intense therapy work she had done, she had accessed more specific details, had slowly pieced together what had happened and, with help, had accomplished a large portion of the difficult healing from this unimaginable agony. Anne still carried a tremendous amount of fear embedded throughout her body, which left her feeling drained and numb. She admitted that she also suffered from numerous addictions that reflected her attempts to self-medicate the fear, pain and memories.

I thanked Anne for sharing her story and told her I was sure we could impact the substantial archived trauma she carried and release it. I gave her a brief overview of how the session would unfold so she would know what to expect. First, I guided her in a grounding exercise, making sure she was present in her physical body in the room, and then asked permission to remove the heavy energy from her aura. I began the cleansing with a Peruvian cologne called *Agua de Florida*, which carries the strong scent of lavender, citrus and amber. I sprayed it over her, head to toe, to remove the initial layer of dense energy. I then used a large, dark wing feather to sweep a second coating layer of energy into the ground. Following the feather, I engaged a black wooden staff to collect the final toxic energy enveloping her aura and discharged it into the ground through my sacred altar.

When I finished this cleansing, Anne reported that she felt lighter already, noting that it was as if a heavy blanket had been lifted from her. Continuing, I guided her in an extraction process to pull additional obstructing energies out of her body, using a 3-inch black tourmaline crystal from my altar. When she completed the extraction, I instructed her in releasing these energies by blowing them forcefully into the ground. Anne was acutely sensitive to the effects of this process and gave me a vivid description of the tarry energies moving down her arm and into my stone.

Anne and I moved on to a guided process for identifying, conversing with and expelling disembodied energetic beings that I sensed were plaguing her. I generally refer to these non-corporeal beings as *entities* or *thought-forms*. One by one, we were able to locate and evict five noxious entities that she was carrying. Each of these was a shadowy, parasitic being that was blocking the flow of energy throughout Anne's physical and energetic bodies, as well as causing her emotional distress. Even though all five had been deeply embedded, she easily expelled them with the help of spirit guides.

There was one more, however, that had been in Anne for a very long time. It was aggressive and hostile, refusing to cooperate. This violent, malevolent being slowly began strangling her as we attempted to remove it. Anne had terrible memories of being strangled, resulting from her childhood ritual abuse, and this action threw her into a panic. Her voice sputtered as she became more alarmed, and I could see she was unable to completely let go of the entity. We quickly enlisted higher guides to help us, and Anne reported that they immediately came into her awareness. She asked them to help her expel this onerous being and reported seeing them remove "most of the creature." We thanked the guides for their rapid assistance, and I made a mental note of this partial removal to address later. Anne said she felt noticeably more spacious—there was more room for her own presence and she felt more at home in her body.

I then described the next process, which I referred to as a guided shamanic journey. Anne said she was ready and opted to lie on a pad beside my altar for this part of our session. I gave her a blanket, a pillow and a blindfold to enhance her comfort and ability to relax. I then assisted her in entering a light trance state, in which she could more easily access her unconscious, and led her down a series of steps and through a gateway into an altered state of awareness. I directed her to call in a higher guide for this journey work. When the spirit being appeared, we ascertained that he was in service of the light and an appropriate guide for the session.

I advised Anne to ask this luminous being to take her to an optimal place for working on her issues. Anne reported that she had been transported somewhere and now seemed to be in a deep fog. She couldn't see anything, nor was she feeling much. I began to feel a vivid somatic sensation of the excising of large amounts of dense, putrid energy from deep in her being. There was no content to go along with these sensations and no story or visions for either of us. I had the strong impression that her angelic guide removed large amounts of highly toxic energy from her body and energy field. My felt sense of this detoxing process persisted for the entire session. I intuited that Anne's spirit helper was purposefully employing this shielded manner of working to spare her the horror of reviewing intense and traumatic details of her torture. I felt this was wise and a profound blessing for Anne, and when I shared my observation with her, she readily agreed.

Gradually, the fog cleared. Anne became aware that she was in a dimly lit natural, forested landscape and was seeing a large rocky outcrop in the distance. I urged her to ask her guide if she had entered a past life, and he conveyed that yes, she was viewing a past-life event. Anne moved toward a clearing near the rocks and reported seeing "scary, witch-like people, wearing masks and dancing around a fire" they had built there. Her attention was then drawn to a cave entrance opposite the fire. A "princess-like person, richly dressed and wearing an ornate headdress" came out of the cave, and Anne knew that the woman was herself in this past life.

Anne continued narrating her encounter. The woman emerged as though in a trance, slowly approached the masked group, and was then securely bound with many coarse ropes by several of the dancers. We were both on pins and needles, apprehensive that something horrific was about to happen when, suddenly, everything went black in Anne's vision. We each clearly sensed that she did not need to re-experience the details of what happened in that past life. The spirit guide confirmed that it was enough to glimpse it and to know that it had happened.

The light being gave Anne specific information concerning the energetic accumulation she still carried from that past life and showed her how this archived energy had influenced much of her experience in this lifetime. I suggested she ask her spirit helper if we could clear this deposit. "Yes," he answered. I asked Anne if she would like to release this harmful cache, and she immediately assented. I then directed her to ask him to facilitate the clearing and heal the toxic energetic charges from this past life. He assured us he would and proceeded to clear and heal it all. Anne was astounded at what she felt happening energetically in her body. She told me she experienced profound physical and emotional relief from this clearing and felt it as deeply sacred healing. She described it as having been encased or coated in multiple dense and ugly layers, and now she was free and clean at last. We then asked the guide to fill the spaces where these energies had been archived with whatever she chose to replace them with. She asked to be filled with love and light.

At this point, I encouraged Anne to ask her guide if there were any fragments or disembodied pieces of herself that we could retrieve at this time. The higher being affirmed that there were lost pieces and immediately took her to a place where she could see "four little lights." Anne said she knew these were parts of herself, even though they appeared to her as nebulous, unformed clouds of energy. I explained that when we experience trauma that we are not able to contain and integrate, a fragment of our being may cleave off, carrying the emotional charge of the event, as well as the memory of it. I told her I had a strong sense that these fragments were from her experience both as a fetus and as a small infant.

Anne replied that she was not receiving any content or story about these lost pieces, yet knew they were essential parts of herself and wanted them back. We asked the spirit being for help, and he gently brought the glowing pieces back to her. Together they reinstated the little lights into her body through her heart chakra. He then performed a further energetic clearing of the fragments once they settled inside her. I urged her to ask if there was anything else that he could return to her at this time. The guide brought forth what Anne described as a small golden ball, which she felt was an energetic gift. He gently placed this ball inside her heart. We both shared the impression that inside the ball were the qualities of faith and hope. Anne said the gift felt miraculous and gratefully received it. She watched as the golden ball dissolved into her body, giving her warm feelings of safety and comfort. We paused for a few moments to let this energy assimilate.

As we continued the journey, Anne gradually realized that she was standing on the edge of a tall, sheer cliff. She recalled an experience when she was younger, where she was standing on a similar rugged cliff face. In her memory, she saw the wind like a living spirit coming to her and speaking with her. I asked if the wind was one of her allies, and she replied with a wistful "Yes." I asked her if she could call on the wind for healing and clearing. "Yes," she said. "I can." We then asked her higher guide if he would be available to teach her more about working with the wind, and he replied that he would be delighted to help her. I encouraged Anne to make this a part of her spiritual practice, to which she happily agreed.

Anne then described being suddenly transported to what appeared to be a surgical suite. She said she was now "feeling numb and brain dead." I sensed that her luminous guide was executing another round of deep spiritual surgery on her. I felt this physically, in my own body, as painful, horrific energy deposits that were being extracted and cleared. This surgery continued for some minutes. When I checked with Anne, she said she had received no content nor story of what had transpired and explained that her experience of it "was like being in deep anesthesia." Once the intense surgery was complete, Anne reported feeling only peace and ease, along with the knowledge that the guide had removed considerable embedded damage.

At this point, I remembered the vile entity that we had not been able to completely evict. I asked Anne to request that the guide help her expel the remaining part of the strangling creature and take it where it belonged. The spirit helper fulfilled this request instantly, thoroughly removing the noxious being from her body. Anne stated that she now felt even more relief and spaciousness, and we both thanked her spirit guide.

The luminous being then advised us that we had done enough work for the day. I told Anne to ask him to please take her back to the gateway where she had begun her journey. I encouraged her to thank this masterful guide again for all he had done for her. He told Anne he would always be available to her, and they agreed to continue the work together now that she was aware he existed and could easily contact him.

When Anne was ready to return, I brought her back up into this, our everyday reality. After a few minutes, she was able to sit, and I was struck by how different she looked. The woman in front of me appeared to be an entirely changed person from the one I had met only hours ago. She was smiling, the deep lines in her face had softened and her skin was rosy; a new lightness had replaced her earlier somber spirit. When I asked how she was feeling, she said she was tired yet felt deeply cleansed, renewed and reborn.

I told Anne that the work we had done would continue to unfold over the next days and weeks, and then taught her how to do energy cleansing and entity removals on her own in case more entities appeared over time. I recommended she perform the cleansing daily and gave her a healing stone from my altar to use for extracting blocking energy. In return, she promised that she would regularly practice these techniques and continue her healing process by working with her spirit guide.

We ended our lengthy session by closing sacred space and thanking our spiritual support team. Her higher guide still felt very present in the room with us, which was unusual yet welcome. It gave us both the feeling that we were powerfully protected, supported and held. Anne thanked me for guiding her through the process and told me she was amazed and deeply grateful for the work that we had done. She was thrilled to have encountered her spirit guide and was eagerly looking forward to working with him in the future. I thanked Anne for having the courage to participate in this intense session. As I walked her to the door, I, too, was filled with gratitude for the profound healing and transformation I had witnessed. Anne was radiant.

Chapter 2

Spiritual Energy Work

WHAT AM I DESCRIBING IN Chapter 1? What do I mean by energy cleansing, entities, the unconscious, past lives, soul fragments and allies? How does healing happen? Is it real? Is it a placebo? Is it fantasy, or wishful thinking? These are all pertinent questions.

The healing methodologies I describe in this book are ancient. They have been used for millennia, then discarded by Western culture, and are now returning. They fall within the broader field of energy healing, including holistic, traditional, folk, shamanic and spiritual approaches. Only recently has energy healing become the subject of scientific research, and it is now gaining wider acceptance. Therapeutic energy work includes a wide variety of techniques that co-operate directly with the body's energy systems on physical, emotional, mental and spiritual levels to restore a person's well-being.

All body systems depend upon the free flow and balance of energy throughout to maintain health. Reiki and acupuncture have been the most studied forms of energy healing. Other widely practiced modalities include acupressure, reflexology, healing touch, Emotional Freedom Technique (or tapping) and qi gong as well as sound, pranic, crystal, quantum and shamanic healing. Some of these are hands-on techniques, and some are not. Some are practiced in person, while others utilize remote healing.

Research continues—mainly from a physical standpoint—attempting to measure and quantify the bio-energy we emit as human beings. I approach energy healing from a spiritual or consciousness-based perspective, which aligns with shamanic and quantum healing modalities. My focus is on engaging beneficent spiritual guides in the nonphysical realms for direct assistance. They perform the actual healing. This methodology contrasts with techniques that apply energy directly to the body or bio-field, also called the aura, using one's hands, tools, or sound.

Ultimately, our physical body is composed of vibration, which is energy and also information. Thus, I believe all healing is essentially energy healing. Humanity is now on the brink of a foundational transformation in healing and healthcare. This transformation requires medicine and healthcare to catch up with current knowledge of consciousness, quantum mechanics and information theory. The words *energy, consciousness,* and *vibration* or *frequency* are basically interchangeable. The latest research into the nature of reality indicates that everything is, at its essence, information. This information is composed of myriad energies, some of which are precursors that lie in a different dimension than our physical universe. I define nonphysical energies as *spiritual* or *quantum energies,* all of which are essentially available to us via the higher guides.

I will use the terms *physical* and *nonphysical* since we are used to thinking in those terms. Our nonphysical/energetic bodies: the emotional, mental and etheric or spiritual bodies form the aura. Traditional cultures understand that it is the intrusion of energies or spirits into the bio-field or body that causes illness. Healing involves removing these obstructing intrusions. Energy practitioners have discovered that much dis-ease arises from unresolved emotional trauma, which becomes embedded or archived as energy deposits in one or more of a person's bodies. These two views are nearly identical. In other words, some form of energy is lodged in a person and blocks health and well-being. There is always an energetic component to every illness. Asking whether these energies are physical, emotional, mental or spiritual is akin to asking whether they are waves or particles.

Once we observe them, they are no longer what they were, as the very acts of viewing and defining them separates them from the whole.

Humans have recognized obstructing energies and removed them from each other since time immemorial. Many methodologies exist for addressing and discharging these embedded energies. The processes presented in this book are modalities that have emerged through my training and healing work over more than forty years, and they continue to transform as my consciousness evolves. Most important, however, is that these techniques are pragmatic. They work. How the healing happens is not as crucial to me as the efficacy. Research may eventually shine a light on the mechanisms at work behind the scenes.

I conduct all sessions with the intention to facilitate the highest level of healing possible for each person. Over time, I have consistently witnessed that the repair, cleansing, clearing and transformations that occur during sessions result in improved wellness for my clients. In other words, real, palpable beneficial change accrues to the individual experiencing this quantum-level energy healing, and these changes persist over time. It is well documented that mystical states of consciousness can produce physical healing in humans. I have observed that they also promote emotional, mental and spiritual healing. The guided shamanic journeys consistently induce mystical-state experiences for the journeyer, as reported by that person.

I use the term *unconscious* to represent the initial destination for these guided journeys. What is the unconscious? How do we know it even exists? The answers to these intriguing questions are wide-ranging and beyond the scope of this book. However, I generally favor Carl Jung's view of the unconscious, with its distinction of personal and collective levels, as a useful working model. In classic shamanism, reality consists of three worlds to which one can journey: the upper, the middle and the lower. The lower world is the unconscious, which is also interior or within. I use the term *unconscious* because it can have more neutral and less challenging connotations than *the lower world*. One does not need to know what the unconscious is to journey there; one only needs to be willing to suspend judgment, go, and experience it directly. Jung also suggests that the experiences we have in the unconscious, whether they are "real" or not, offer great wisdom for healing and personal growth.

We each have our own ideas, beliefs, cosmology and ways of understanding what we think constitutes reality. We also know that we, as humans, are seeing a minuscule slice of what actually exists. Western culture emphasizes and values the physical as the only reality—or at least the only relevant reality. This bias apparently arose from the separation of science from religion during the Middle Ages, thus splitting the physical from the spiritual. As a result, Western culture has developed dysfunctional behaviors concerning the rest of creation, which remains unified. This impairment has been particularly acute in our conventional medical education and practice with its myopic view of reality.

The aberrant belief in the separation of spirit from matter is slowly changing as we attempt to catch up to both ancient and current ways of understanding reality. Ancient wisdom traditions tell us that all physical reality first exists as potentiality in the nonphysical or spiritual realms, and then emerges into this world of form. Modern physics supports this view, as Jude Currivan, PhD, explains in her book, *The Cosmic Hologram*: "… nothing in our Universe is ultimately random; everything that manifests in the physical world emerges from deeper and ordered levels of nonphysical and in-formed reality."[1]

Additionally, we now know that physical matter makes up only about 5% of the physical universe. The majority, based on current estimates, includes 27% dark matter and some 68% dark energy. What are dark matter and dark energy? Could they be other forms of consciousness?

Embedded energetic charges within the unconscious dominate our psyches, our bodies and even our DNA until we clear them. We are now discovering the mechanisms by which emotional energy exerts an effect at the physical level. When we bring this material buried in the unconscious into our awareness, we can make beneficial choices that lead us toward healing. How can these embedded charges be cleared? What might be an effective mechanism?

Spiritual wisdom states that higher vibration always lifts up and dismantles that which is lower vibration. This wisdom is known as "spiritual law" and is the reason for employing higher guides in healing, as they manifest spiritual law. How does this healing occur? At our current level of consciousness, we are unable to understand the answer to this question. This reminds me of Arthur C. Clarke's statement, "Any sufficiently advanced technology is indistinguishable from magic."[2] In this case, the advanced technology is consciousness or Spirit.

There is a great deal that we humans do not fully comprehend. Electricity and gravity are two examples that come to mind. However, we still use a working model of many of these not-yet-understood natural phenomena to our advantage. My lack of understanding of how these energy healing modalities work adds a dimension of delight and wonder to the sessions. Coming from a shamanic perspective, I see my role in facilitating the healing techniques as an interface between Spirit, the Great Mystery or the quantum field and the person seeking healing. I am a bridge of consciousness between different manifestations of reality, not the one doing the healing. Spirit is the source of the information and energies received by the client. I function more as a tour guide and catalyst for the journey into other realities.

* * *

Ruth was a silver-haired woman approaching retirement from her corporate job, and also worked as an energy healer. I had known her for quite some time before she decided to ask me for help. I queried her about the issue she wanted to address, and she disclosed that, for as long as she could remember, she had been unable to speak her truth. This blockage was most acute, she said, whenever she was in a challenging situation with someone of authority. She was very eager to heal this condition, and I told her we could most likely get right to the crux of this issue.

Ruth and I met in her comfortable living room, where I had set up a small, portable altar that honored the seven sacred directions and the natural elements. Standing before the altar, we began by opening sacred space and inviting in our spiritual support. Ruth said she felt a definite shift in the room as we did this. I proceeded with a series of three energy cleansings using floral waters, feathers and an empowered staff to sweep the obstructing energy from her aura into the ground. We then sat down on her roomy sofa, and I guided her in the process of expelling entities. She succeeded in contacting and removing several of these beings and sent them on with their guides. I asked if she felt she could do this process by herself since more entities might emerge over time, and she was confident she could.

Following this, I gave Ruth an overview of the guided shamanic journey, along with the option to sit up or lie down for it. She chose to sit up, resting comfortably on the sofa. I closed the shades to darken the room and, using progressive relaxation to deepen her state, led her down a flight of steps into the unconscious. Once she had walked through the stone gateway, I directed her to call in a higher guide for the journey. We ascertained that this light being was appropriate for the session, so I asked her to request that the spirit helper allow her to experience the source of her difficulty in speaking her truth.

Immediately, Ruth found herself in a shocking scene. She felt that she was in a past life looking at a dead woman hanging—rope around her neck—from a tree branch. We asked for clarification, and the higher guide confirmed that this was Ruth in a previous life. When we requested more information, he conveyed that this woman had been hanged as a witch for speaking her truth. In that lifetime, the woman's truth was considered blasphemy, and she was executed. As difficult as it was for Ruth to witness this scene, it uncovered a real answer to her question. What was striking to me was that the woman was still hanging from the tree. It indicated that her energy had been trapped, or frozen, in that moment of death and was still there.

When I voiced my feelings to Ruth, she agreed. I urged her to ask the spirit being what we could do to clear and repair this energetic archive, both from the past life and from Ruth's current one. He directed Ruth to cut the body of her former self down from the tree, remove the rope, and make the body ready for burial. This process was lovingly assisted by the spirit guide, who then opened a grave in the soft earth near the tree. I encouraged Ruth to prepare, anoint and dress the body in any way she wanted.

With gentleness and loving-kindness, she placed the body in the grave. We both participated in a spontaneous ceremony to release this deceased self. Ruth said many prayers and took some time to grieve this experience. She then filled the grave with flowers, sang and rattled over it. When she had finished, the higher being covered the grave and told Ruth that the past life, and its attendant trauma, were now healed. We requested that he safely transport the woman's energy to the spirit realm, which the luminous being then confirmed he had done. Ruth had not been aware that she had been carrying anything but now said she felt as if a proverbial millstone had been lifted from around her neck. Then she added that the shock of seeing this gruesome death had also been released, and she felt a pervading sense of closure, serenity and peace. I told her I felt a sense of great relief as well.

I directed Ruth to inquire about other past lives where she was not allowed to speak her truth. She asked and instantly found herself in another previous life in which she had also been a wise woman and a healer. She watched in horror as she witnessed her past-life self, a young woman in a long, flowing dress, being tied to a tall pole in a large, grassy clearing, surrounded by an anxious mob of people. We were both filled with trepidation as the woman was about to be burned alive. The guide told her that, in this past life, she had written many books about healing and nature. These books now surrounded her as fuel where she was bound. Again, Ruth realized that she was about to be killed for speaking—and writing—her truth.

As Ruth watched the lighting of the fire, we asked what we could do to clear and heal this lifetime. The higher guide directed Ruth to rescue her former self from the fire. She reached into the flames, pulled the woman out of the fire and brought her close. This response was novel and surprising.

My experiences had, up to that moment, all been after the fact, clearing and healing death trauma. This woman, inexplicably, was not dead. We could only accept the experience and proceed with the journey as it unfolded. I had the sudden insight that this woman possessed a priceless gift for Ruth. Clearly, she did not have a problem with speaking her truth.

We asked the spirit being if we could bring this aspect of Ruth's former self, with her developed attribute of speaking her truth, into her current incarnation. The guide replied, "Of course!" He prompted Ruth to talk to her past self, explaining that she was this same woman in a future lifetime. She told the woman that she wanted her to come into this current life and be a part of her. Ruth's past self quickly comprehended this request and excitedly agreed to join her.

With the help of the higher guide, Ruth gathered up the energies of this past self and incorporated them into her heart chakra. As this happened, she told me all of it gently integrated into her body, mind and spirit, and she felt a new, expansive sense of herself opening up. Both Ruth and I were completely surprised by this. We each had guided many people in soul retrievals over the years. Neither of us, however, had even conceived of performing a soul retrieval from a past life. We paused for a while to let this experience integrate.

Continuing, we asked the higher being if there were any other soul retrievals we could enact from either past or present lives. He carried Ruth to what appeared to be a cluster of fragments. She described them as a constellation of energies, and her guide informed us that these had all split off in her current lifetime, during childhood. We inquired whether they needed to return individually or if the spirit being could recover them as a group. He assisted Ruth in scooping them all up and bringing them into her body via her solar plexus. Once there, they began to reintegrate smoothly into her body. I reminded her of the importance of caring for these recovered aspects of herself, giving her examples of ways to accomplish this.

When I finished the instruction, the guide advised us that we had completed our session. I directed Ruth to request that he return her to the gateway, where she had begun her journey, and prompted her to thank him for the incredible healing he had facilitated. The spirit helper promised to be available to her for future endeavors, and she expressed her desire to continue to work with him.

When Ruth was ready, I brought her back up the steps into the reality of the everyday world. She was in awe of her guide and exhilarated by her journey experiences. Even though it had been intense, painful and even shocking, it all made total sense to her. She smiled as she told me she felt both relieved and grateful not only to have answered her question but to have cleared and healed her past. With child-like glee, she again said she was delighted to have her new spirit guide. She felt deeply fulfilled by all she had experienced and was looking forward to reconnecting to the many recovered aspects of herself. I felt honored to witness the profound healing facilitated by her higher guide and told her she looked much more alive. We talked for a long time, allowing her to integrate more of her feelings. To end our session, we thanked our spiritual support team and closed sacred space.

A few weeks later, I got a call from a jubilant Ruth. She had just been in a situation at work that involved challenging comments her boss had made to her. In the past, she would not have been able to speak her truth by stating her conflicting point of view. She proudly reported that this time she had been able to say what she needed to, with confidence, clarity and calmness. She said she felt more whole and now had a stronger sense of herself. We were both elated with this outcome.

Chapter 3

Spirit Guides and Healing

MY PRIMARY HEALING MODALITY IS the guided shamanic journey, in which I guide a person through an experience in the imaginal realm. The term *imaginal* refers to the world of images. This concept contrasts with our usual idea of imagining something because the word *imagination* typically implies that things are unreal, fabricated or fantasy. This shamanic journey could also be called a nonphysical journey, travel into non-ordinary reality, or an altered state of consciousness. It is different from classical shamanic journeys since the main focus is to connect my client to one (or more) of their spiritual guides, who will then facilitate the healing endeavor. It also contrasts with many other hands-on energy healing approaches, and especially other shamanistic journey techniques that are currently taught.

The modalities presented in this book rely on the participation of the individual who is seeking healing. It is this participation, I believe, that guarantees the healing received will be potent and lasting for that person. In many Indigenous traditions, the one seeking healing must take an active part in the healing for it to be deemed successful. Each client I work with connects directly with their spirit guide, actively requests the restorative actions, and personally experiences the entire interactive session. Participation is the foundation of this work.

Successful client outcomes depend on two basic conditions. First, the person must genuinely want to heal and be willing to face the unknown. Secondly, they must have the capacity to do this type of imaginal journey work, which can be experienced through any combination of our senses. Never has a client returned from their guided journey wondering if anything really happened or questioning the results. Each person knows and remembers what they experienced, understands it firsthand, and is empowered by it. The experiences are rarely nebulous and never theoretical.

Higher light beings oversee the therapeutic work, so there is no danger that it will be inappropriate or harmful to either the client or practitioner. The celestial guides and the individual's psyche orchestrate the journey content, delineate the work to be done and accomplish the healing. I do not dictate or determine the client's experience. Nor do I lead the person toward specific events, or treat/cure any ailments; this sets these techniques apart from other healing modalities.

Wisdom teachers from ancient times tell us that all healing is done by the person themselves, with the help of Spirit. In some traditions, it is improper for anyone to call themselves a healer because it is seen as dishonest and disrespectful of Spirit. I do not consider myself a healer, even though clients coming from a conventional medical paradigm may expect someone else to heal them. For the techniques presented here, the practitioner functions as a guide, a coach and a facilitator who oversees the session and holds the energetic container for the healing. Most salient, in my opinion, is that it is the client who directly requests the healing, and it is this request that allows the spirit beings to accomplish their tasks. My service as a conduit between Spirit and human beings fosters energy work that is clean and straightforward.

The healing techniques are designed to be implemented in a client-practitioner model or, in other words, working as a pair. To me, this embodies the current re-emerging paradigm of the Divine Feminine. When we work in pairs, we become a team, focused on cooperation, collaboration and sharing. The team then opens to include spirit realm helpers, in their myriad forms, to generate healing. These modalities are inclusive and focus on connection, building relationships, and the unity, balance and harmony of all things. These are primary qualities of the Divine Feminine. The invitation of spirit guides and requests for their assistance opens the field to a virtually unlimited energetic resource—the quantum field. Our acknowledgment of the realms of Spirit demonstrates our understanding that all beings are connected and that, ultimately, we are all One Consciousness.

We humbly recognize that our human ability to address the emotional, mental, spiritual and energetic basis of debilitating conditions is crude and limited. However, for illumined beings, these are simple matters. Spirit guides have communicated that they reside in a state where they are everyone, everywhere, at the same time, and thus know everything. In other words, they are in Unity Consciousness. The emerging cooperative paradigm starkly contrasts to our current cultural focus on separation, control, exclusivity, manipulation and power over other humans and nature. Humanity's relentless dissection of the whole into smaller and smaller pieces has now taken us to the quantum realization that there is no separation. All things are conjoined at the smallest levels of the physical Universe and thus at every level. The Western world's relentless dissection process, along with our subject-object form of language, has resulted in the fragmentation of human awareness. It is the measurement itself that breaks the Oneness into parts.

The healing work outlined here recognizes and aligns with the complementary dualism from which physical creation is born. This cosmology is expressed most beautifully in the Taoist symbol of the yin and the yang. Everything is contained within the whole and manifests as complementary dual forms, with everything connected to everything else and within an eternal flow. Each complementary aspect also contains within it the seed of its opposite in the eternal dance of being. There is no separation—there is only inextricable complementarity. Dualism is part and parcel of our perceived reality on the physical plane. Opposites, such as positive and negative, combine to make a whole. As many spiritual teachers have taught, duality represents the two sides of a single coin. The coin is the indivisible whole, of which two apparent sides are opposite and complementary. The goal is to restore the balance and harmony of the whole upon which all healing rests.

The reader will notice that I repeat the instructions for opening sacred space and calling in spiritual support, as well as closing the session, in every case study. This repetition is important to the entrainment of these techniques in the student. These steps are crucial and cannot be skipped.

* * *

Ellen, whom I did not know, emailed to ask about my healing work. She explained that she had listened to a webcast on shamanism and healing and as a result of what she heard, decided she needed shamanic healing. Ellen admitted that she had had no idea where to find a shaman but, serendipitously, happened to see a flyer posted in her community co-op. The flyer announced a workshop on shamanism that I would be teaching the following month. Ellen asked if I did individual healing work. I told her I did not consider myself a shaman but would be willing to do energy healing work with her. I gave her the date and times I would be available on the weekend of the workshop. We corresponded, setting the appointment and briefly discussing her background and health issues.

At the appointed time, Ellen came in to meet me in a wheelchair. She could not walk. Her arms were turned in on themselves somewhat like unopened ferns. Her hair was a dull brown, her complexion grey, and her voice was barely above a whisper due to a large goiter in her neck. Ellen reiterated that she had many medical problems that left her with no energy and that each of these conditions was rapidly getting worse. She had tried many kinds of allopathic and alternative healing, yet none had been able to impact the causes of her dis-ease. At this point, Ellen was depressed and in despair. She had recently concluded that all her conditions were spiritually based, which was why she wanted to see me.

I was surprised by Ellen's drastic appearance and wondered what I could do for her. Instantly, I remembered that Spirit had brought her to me, and Spirit would do the healing. I greeted Ellen and wheeled her in front of my sacred altar. She spent a few minutes taking in the energy of the room and everything in it. She commented that she liked the symmetry, beauty, balance and energy of my altar with all the colorful crystals and artifacts. I told her she was free to explore it if it called to her.

I began the session by explaining what it would entail, and Ellen agreed to participate as best she could. We opened sacred space together and called in our spiritual support, which she greatly enjoyed. I performed a series of energetic cleansings of her aura using spicy, fragrant water, a feather and my black wooden staff as she sat in her wheelchair. She was highly sensitive and able to feel the nonphysical energies being removed and discharged, and remarked that she felt lighter with each cleansing.

Following that, I handed Ellen the tourmaline crystal from my altar and explained that she would use it to extract more impeding energies from her body. She fully immersed herself in this process. When finished, she said she felt a large amount of thick, heavy energy leaving her body and going into the stone—even stating that the stone became very heavy in the process. I then guided her to clear the stone by transferring these obstructing energies into the ground via my altar. I asked her if she thought she could do extractions on her own. When she said she could, I offered her a stone from my altar to use at home and suggested that she repeat the extraction steps every week. She thanked me for the gift and readily agreed to do them.

I knew Ellen was carrying entities. I explained my understanding of these beings and what they can do in a person's body. She said she understood this and felt she had several entities but didn't know what to do to get them out. I outlined the removal process we would use, and we began. Ellen was empathic, psychically gifted and able to communicate clearly with each creature. One by one, as I guided her, she located and addressed half a dozen entities. All of these beings were malevolent and entrenched in her body. With the combined help of her guides and Archangel Michael, we were able to remove each one and have it permanently taken away. We discussed her being extremely empathic, open and sensitive, and the importance of having good boundaries. I explained what is meant by this term and how she could maintain them. She confided that this had always been a nebulous idea for her. I admitted that it had been a difficult concept for me also.

Next, I outlined the guided shamanic journey and asked Ellen if she had concerns before we began. She replied that she was ready to go and sat calmly in her wheelchair as I led her down the steps into the unconscious and through the gateway. When I directed her to call in her higher guide, she reported that both Archangels Michael and Raphael came into her vision. I suggested she ask if they were the guides to facilitate the healing work. She told me they said, "No, we are the Overseers," and with that, a smaller angel appeared. We determined that this angel was the appropriate light-filled guide for the journey.

Ellen had previously confided that she was sure her autoimmune disease had a spiritual cause. She also had severe osteoarthritis that she felt was from Spirit. I directed her to ask her angel to take her to the inception of her autoimmune issues. She reported immediately finding herself in front of a large, dark cave entrance in an unknown land. She described the scene as filled with a horde of people wearing medieval clothing. They all had torches, and many small fires were burning in a wide semicircle in front of the cave. I urged her to confirm with her spirit guide that this was a past life, and his response was affirmative.

Ellen told me she knew she was there to witness something. Slowly, she realized that she was there to observe the sacrifice of her daughter. As she related this to me, the memory of that lifetime flooded into her, and she broke down in sobs. I could feel the trauma energy pouring off of her as she witnessed this scene in great detail. We paused for a few minutes to allow her to feel the impact of this experience. The angel imparted to her that the purpose of re-experiencing this event was twofold: she needed to know that this energy was from a past-life incident and the remembering of it also served as an initiation in her current life. I encouraged her to submit to the entirety of this phenomenon as fully as possible and gave her time and space to do it.

The luminous guide then told Ellen she needed to scream out her feelings to heal the sizable goiter in her neck. She questioned me about screaming, and I replied that it was safe to let it out. I urged her to put 100 percent into the scream. She shrieked and wailed loudly for several minutes, and I encouraged her to keep going until she felt she had released all the archived energy. Her screaming finally tapered off and then stopped. She was exhausted.

At that point, I felt inspired to give Ellen a description of the wounded healer archetype. This archetype pertains to one who has experienced pain on a very deep level, has learned how to heal their own wounds, and then uses this wisdom to transmute suffering and pain into healing for others. As I moved through this explanation, she told me her angelic guide began showing her images of wounded healers, which underscored my narrative. She said these images impacted her profoundly and that old, stuck energies were flowing off her into the ground. I intuited that she needed to take some action to catalyze this archetypal transmutation and suggested she could take her initiation to the next level by opening an energy portal into her new life as a healer. Not missing a beat, Ellen opened a luminous portal in her journey reality. As she did this, I felt a powerful energy shift and recommended that she complete her transformation by walking through this doorway into her new life.

As Ellen imagined herself stepping through the portal, I perceived her moving into a shower of grace and blessings from the celestial realms. I told her what I was feeling, and she replied that she could not express in words what she was experiencing. We let this blessing integrate for a few minutes more. I told her what I had seen and that extensive healing had happened in the higher planes. It will precipitate, I continued, down through the levels until it comes into manifestation in your physical body, which will then transform. Her higher guide confirmed that this was happening as we spoke. We then talked for many minutes, as she asked me numerous questions about her experience.

The angel then announced we had done enough for one day, and I directed Ellen to request that her guide return her to the gateway. She thanked the spirit being and the two overseeing archangels, and they all departed. She told me she now understood that these beings always were, and would always be, available to her whenever she called upon them. For Ellen, knowing that she was continuously held by Spirit made an enormous difference. She then indicated she was ready to return, and I brought her up the steps into our everyday reality.

Once Ellen was present in the room, she began crying again. She was overwhelmed and shaken by the enormity of her journey. After a few minutes, she became calm and centered as new life began flowing through her. I then performed a series of energetic empowerments, using high-vibration floral waters and a large feather to fill her aura with fortifying energies and prayers. We had a long conversation to help integrate her intense episode. Ellen was smiling as she said she understood that her life experiences are all part of her healer's path. I confirmed what she was saying, phrasing it as on-the-job training that all those on the path experience. Ellen stated that she was committed to her spiritual growth, no matter what, and I congratulated her on her courage and commitment to healing. Before we closed, I ensured that she could enact all the processes we had employed during the session. Ellen replied that she understood them and was confident she could continue the work by herself, with assistance from her angelic spirit guides. I told her I believed that she could.

We thanked our spiritual support and closed sacred space. When I again looked at Ellen, I saw that her face and body were full of healthy color, and the grey cast was entirely gone. Her eyes were shining, she was smiling, and there was a vibrant life-force energy about her. She was sitting straighter in her wheelchair, her body held upright, and was animatedly gesturing and talking in a normal voice about her experiences. She told me that, even though she knew the work with me would be transforming, she was astounded at how extensive the session was for her. She began to cry again, this time with tears of gratitude for all that had been removed and healed. I agreed that this had been a surprisingly powerful session and that it was, in part, due to her courage in facing the unknown. She thanked me for taking the time to see her and for the healing I had facilitated. As

I wheeled her to the door where her friend awaited, I told her I was sure she would be a phenomenal healing practitioner.

* * *

Indigenous elders stress the importance of creating an integral container for all healing work. What does it mean to have "an integral container?" What's a container? It is a term used in psychotherapy yet also applies to energy healing. Jung introduced the concept of containing the therapy process. He likened it to that of alchemy, in which a container was necessary to safely hold all elements so that they could interact and transform. The process involves providing a protective, sacred place where all feelings, thoughts, experiences and potentials are welcome, respected and available to the alchemical healing process.

There are many techniques for creating and then opening sacred space, which is intrinsic to the container and a prerequisite for any sincere healing endeavor. The method employed to open the sacred space is not as important as the authenticity with which it is enacted. This quote from Tanya Wilkinson, PhD, summarizes the role of the container: "Successful access to the transformative power of the unconscious requires an adequate container; the cauldron must have sturdy sides to withstand the chaos of regeneration."[3] To reach the deepest levels of healing, there must be equivalent levels of safety, trust, honesty, respect and compassion between the parties involved. High integrity, focused intention and alignment with Spirit are essential.

Many ancient cultures, and all original peoples, know that everything that exists is alive. Whether animal, plant, stone, physical or nonphysical, all is energy, all is vibration. Everything is also conscious, interconnected and in communication with itself. The nonphysical, energetic or spiritual realms are teeming with life forms, beings, consciousness and information, much of which we may call upon for assistance and healing. In my experience, every being has at least one guide who is willing to be of service. If multiple spirit beings come forward, one must enlist the most impeccable higher guide to ensure optimum results.

Some cultures recognize "God-given" illness—that which a person has elected to experience as part of their life plan before they incarnate. With these conditions, the individual must find their own way to healing. As I have mentioned, individuals with incurable diseases might be able to obtain deep insight into their illness, the purpose it serves and how they might heal or transform it through speaking with their higher guides. If an individual can participate in the guided journey, there is no downside to exploring restorative options by utilizing the methods presented here.

* * *

Susan, a slender and lively young woman with short blonde hair, was a student in one of my shamanic studies workshops. She was exceptionally sensitive to spiritual energies and asked if I would work with her on some of her past lives. She strongly felt that past-life issues were interfering and blocking her from freely following her purpose in this incarnation. After class one day, we decided to investigate and began with a discussion about her childhood. She revealed that she had experienced a series of abdominal surgeries to remove many tumors and still had daily residual pain. She intuitively sensed the surgeries had left significant trauma embedded in her body, which I agreed was certain. Furthermore, she felt the tumors were connected to some past lives and was very eager to heal those old issues. I told her I would be happy to guide her to uncover the story behind the tumors.

We opened sacred space and called in our spiritual support to assist us. I gave Susan a description of what the session would entail and then commenced with the series of energy cleansings, removing many layers of congested, dense energies from her aura and discharging them into the ground.

Next, Susan and I discussed entities, which I explained are common in people who have had surgery. I posed a series of questions about her physical, emotional and mental states, and her answers allowed her to uncover one entity after another. As I guided her in the entity removal process, she skillfully evicted six sinister beings. All of these were parasitic, blocking the flow of energy through her physical and energetic bodies. She disclosed that she had already removed many other entities over the years in work she had done with spiritual healers. I remarked that I was not surprised and asked whether she felt confident in her ability to do the removal process, should more entities surface. She assured me that she could and would do it.

Following this, I gave Susan an overview of the guided shamanic journey we would do next. She chose to lie down and, when she was comfortable and ready, I led her down into the unconscious. Once she was through the gateway, I prompted her to call in her higher guide. A being she described as full of light appeared in her vision. We determined that this being was genuinely of the light and was the proper guide for the journey.

I directed Susan to tell the spirit being everything she wanted to work on in her journey. When she did so, he whisked her back into one of her childhood surgeries. She was simultaneously on the operating table and observing the scene from a doorway, where she watched the surgeon remove a large number of tumors from her abdomen. Once he removed them, I recommended she ask her guide to show her the actual source of these tumors. In an instant, she found herself in what appeared to be a past life in ancient Egypt. She explained that she saw herself as a young girl who had suffered from the same kinds of tumors. I instructed her to ask if we needed to know more about these tumors in her previous life. The spirit being answered that it was enough for her to see where they had originated. This revelation confirmed her intuition about the source of her tumors being from a past life.

I encouraged Susan to ask if her guide could clear the energetic archive from that lifetime so that it no longer affected her current incarnation. He replied that this was possible, and she asked him to please remove all the tumor energies of this past life. He immediately cleared it all, and she revealed that she felt an extensive energetic shift in her physical body, as if some large, oppressive template had been deleted. She then asked him to fill the void created by the tumor removal with light.

A few moments later, Susan asked the luminous being to completely clear all embedded trauma from the surgeries she had endured in this lifetime. As he began, she told me she could feel the guide restructuring and restoring her peritoneal tissues and organs until all the damage had been repaired. After he finished this extensive clearing, he filled all her tissues and organs with vibrant, healthy energy. Again, she described acutely feeling this happening deep in her physical body, which surprised her. We paused for a few minutes, allowing her to feel and integrate these sensations and healing energies. I told her I applauded her willingness to address this archived distress.

At this point, I suggested that Susan ask the luminous being if there were additional past lives that we could heal. He immediately led her through an entire series of them, which she viewed in succession. One was very intense, and she wanted to tell me about it. She had been a powerful healer who had been "captured, experimented on, tortured, disempowered and manipulated to capture [her] psychic gifts so [she] could be controlled." I agreed that this represented considerable stored trauma that likely affected her current life, and suggested she ask that it be cleared and replaced with whatever she chose. Momentarily, she replied that her guide had completed the removal and was filling her with light, insight and wholeness.

Susan said she had also vividly witnessed and recovered a great many memories of her forgotten Lemurian lifetimes. I urged her to ask if the spirit being could restore more of her memories to allow her to learn from them in her present life. When she asked, he replied, "It has been completed." I then suggested she ask if he could also reinstate her knowledge of her incarnational purpose for this lifetime and how she could fulfill it. He replied that he could and, at her request, he installed this knowledge into her body in the form of a small golden packet. The higher guide explained that this knowledge would "unfold in your life in Divine right timing," and she thanked him for this precious gift.

Following this, I prompted Susan to ask if she could receive shielding and protection in this life, given her extreme sensitivity. "Yes," replied the spirit helper, and he inserted a glowing sapphire crystal into her solar plexus. Susan said she watched as the sapphire completely dissolved into her body. I suggested asking if there was a gift of power that could help her on her path. She reported that the higher being brought forth a large magic staff covered in runes and encrusted with gemstones. He presented it to her and instructed her to use it to restore and re-energize the Earth's grid system. The guide explained that she should use it at Earth power spots to reinstate the energetic balance and harmony of our planet. Susan felt exhilarated as, in great detail, she described the radiant magical gift to me. I asked if she knew how to use this extraordinary staff, and she replied that she did. As she continued to admire it, she announced her intention to start working with it the very next day.

Moments later, the spirit guide let us know we were at the end of the journey. I told Susan to ask him to return her to the gateway, and she reported that she was instantly there. I recommended she ask the higher being if he would be available for further journey work with her. He assured her that he would always be with her and that they could continue working together. I reminded her to thank him for all that he had done, which she happily did. I then led her up the steps into our consensual reality and gave her time to integrate her profound experiences.

Susan was amazed that she felt absolutely transformed by her journey, and said she was filled with beautiful, empowering energies. I told her I could attest that she was, in fact, glowing and radiant. She was thrilled about the gift of her new magic staff and was quite eager to use it. I said I was excited as well, because we do need her to balance and restore the Earth's grid system. She stated that she had already made plans for where she would be using it, starting first thing the next morning.

Susan's face was markedly softer and smoother, and she looked years younger. When I asked about her current level of pain, she replied with surprise that she was no longer in any pain at all. I told her I was happy to hear it and remarked that she looked like she had released a very heavy burden. She agreed and sincerely thanked me for guiding her in such powerful healing work. We were both basking in feelings of gratitude as we closed sacred space and thanked our spiritual support.

Chapter 4

Cosmology and Energy Cleansings

COSMOLOGY IS A WAY OF picturing, or understanding, the cosmos. My use of the term involves both the physical and nonphysical aspects. Coming from a background in mysticism and shamanism, I had numerous experiences of the multiverse—the infinite realms of being that exist all around us. Over time, a working cosmology of the spiritual realms, their configurations and their inhabitants emerged that I found useful in my energy healing practice. I do not think my cosmology is more accurate than any other; I use it because of its empirical practicality. After decades of experience and interaction with nonphysical beings and energies, it simply became normal for me to collaborate with them.

Who or what are the higher guides? How do they know what to do? Who determines which guides appear? I suspect we are a long way from being able to answer these questions. All spiritual traditions have nonphysical denizens: gods, goddesses, guides, saints, prophets, totems, animal allies, ancestors or other categories of spiritual inhabitants. These include a vast array of beings such as elementals, nature spirits and devas, and continue up to the Ascended Masters, saints, Chohans, angels, archangels, extra- and ultra-terrestrial beings and more. I envision spirit beings existing within a matrix of consciousness organized by frequency or vibration, within the

Mind of All That Is. Being in the third-dimensional matrix, we are in one of the lowest, densest and least conscious realms.

I've witnessed that most people can perceive and communicate, to some extent, with countless sentient spiritual beings existing in our shared realities. Incarnated humans have physical and nonphysical bodies, in addition to our higher selves, souls and even higher spiritual aspects. These selves have their existence in the Mind of the Creator, which is also the quantum field. The following quote from Nobel Prize-winning theoretical physicist Max Planck shares this understanding: "All matter originates and exists only by virtue of a force…. We must assume behind this force the existence of a conscious and intelligent Mind. This Mind is the matrix of all matter."[4] Quantum potential is now known to be this underlying intelligence. Since all existence is within the Creator's Mind, we, as part of that Mind, may be able to access unlimited wisdom for healing and the evolution of consciousness.

It is the practitioner's primary responsibility to ensure that the client receives the highest level of healing possible. It is not enough to set sacred space and call in spiritual support and higher guides. The quality of these spirit guides is critical, and it is essential to understand that not just any spirit being will do. The state of being disembodied or spiritual does not ensure that a particular being will be helpful, knowledgeable, or trustworthy. Inhabitants of the lower astral plane, for example, can be clueless. Therefore, it is crucial to verify that one is working with light beings of the highest integrity, capacity, intention and love.

We can classify spiritual beings as either beneficent (expansive) or malevolent (contractive). In other words, they can be thought of as either being "of the light" or "not of the light" when it comes to energy healing work. Partnering solely with beneficent beings who affirm their alignment with Divine Light ensures the best outcome for all concerned.

In my experience over the past four decades, the presence and persistence of dark, contractive spirit beings have increased dramatically in recent years. When I questioned my guides about this, the reply was, "As the light evolves, so does the dark." And an understanding of the unimaginably exquisite energetic balance maintained by the Universe came into my awareness. Currently, I observe that unfavorable beings often appear first when a client calls for a higher guide and that they are more crafty, deceptive and cunning than they used to be. Since this was not the case in the past, I now feel it is essential to evaluate every spirit guide, no matter how they appear.

* * *

Energy Cleansing Process
Overview:

Numerous healing traditions recognize nonphysical, subtle or spiritual energies and beings as sources of illness or health. Shamanic cultures worldwide emphasize the importance of removing harmful energies to restore wellness. Many people can feel, sense, see or even smell these harmful energies in the aura or biofield. Frequently, they appear thick, heavy, opaque and dense and can block or impede the natural flow of healthy energies in our auras and bodies.

Fortunately, anyone who has the intention can usually remove these impeding energies. A practitioner can use any number of substances or tools to sweep the unwanted energies off a person and into the ground. Most commonly, the materials used are the smoke of various plants and resins such as sage, cedar and other herbs as well as copal, myrrh and *palo santo;* floral waters such as colognes, rue and essential oil blends; and tools such as feather fans, *chacapas*, staffs, drums, whistles, rattles, crystals and meteorites. If these tools are not available, you can use your hands to perform the same function.

Contaminating energy is also somewhat fluid, meaning it can flow from one person to another. Thus, it is important to send these energies into the ground to discharge them and not just sweep them off into the environs. There is a distinction between *cleansings* and *clearings*. Cleansing removes the unhealthful energy from a person's aura, while a clearing focuses on the actual source or cause of the issue and heals it. In the energy healing work presented here, clearing is nearly always performed by the higher guides.

There are many sources of contaminating energies: thoughts and emotions we pick up in the process of living our lives; emotional and mental energies directed at us by others; and energies we generate or attract by our thoughts, actions and feelings. These can accumulate in the aura, impeding the free flow of healthy energy. In shamanic cultures, practitioners perceive that harmful energies slowly penetrate the layers of the aura, eventually entering the physical body where they cause physical illness. Therefore, it is optimal to remove these energies when they are still in the aura since once they are inside the body, cleansing is no longer effective in removing them.

I recommend completing a series of cleansings on your client at the beginning of your session, immediately after opening sacred space with them. Always ask your client for permission to cleanse their aura. Ideally, you will perform these in the vicinity of your sacred altar or another focal area for the healing activities. All materials used should be of the highest quality and treated with respect. There are dozens of ways to perform cleansings, and each practitioner will develop their unique style of enacting them. The practitioner must also be attentive to cleansing their own aura. Optimally, this is done both before and after meeting with a client, or a minimum of once per day. The following is one example of a simple three-step cleansing series that can serve as a good beginning.

Step-by-step process:

1. Cleansing with smoke: with your client standing and facing you, light a dried herbal bundle to make the first cleansing pass of the aura with smoke.

   Using your intention to cleanse blocking energies from the aura and deposit them into the ground, start at the top of their head. Moving the smoking bundle back and forth horizontally in a sweeping motion, gradually work your way down the front of the body to the ground. Then have the client turn around and cleanse the back of the body/aura in the same way. If using smoke presents a problem, floral waters in a spray bottle, used in the same manner, can substitute for the herbal bundle.

2. Cleansing with feathers: with the client again facing you, use a single feather, feather fan or bird wing to sweep through their energy field.

   Again, starting at the head, use your intention as you sweep from head to toe, pushing the undesirable energy into the ground. Do this on both the front and back of your client's aura. If you don't have access to or choose not to use these tools, you can vividly imagine doing the cleansing or ask your higher guide to accomplish it for you.

3. Cleansing with light: with your client again facing you, direct them to cleanse themselves with celestial light.

   Ask them to imagine as vividly as possible that they are standing under a waterfall of celestial light. You can assist the client by describing this light and asking them to imagine the light entering their entire physical body and energy field, sweeping all discordant energies into the ground. Suggesting that the client also ask the light to cleanse them augments the process.

4. You may choose to do one or several cleansings. After completing the cleansing, move on to the next process you want to use.

* * *

Jeff was a middle-aged professional who attended one of my shamanic studies workshops. He told me that he loved to go hiking in the mountains and spent a lot of time in nature, but every time he found himself on a high cliff, he felt a compelling urge to throw himself off. He wanted to find the cause of this destructive impulse and heal it—but despite his best efforts, he had made no progress. He asked if I could help him uncover the cause of his disturbing compulsion. I told him we would go into the shamanic journey and see what we could discover.

After calling in our spiritual support, aligning with our highest good and opening sacred space, we began the session. I conducted a series of energy cleansings using floral waters, aromatic smoke, and various other tools from my altar. After completing those, I instructed Jeff in removing extraneous energies using the black tourmaline stone from my altar. He was able to extract considerable unfavorable energy from his body, which he then discharged into the ground with his breath.

Next, we engaged in the entity removal process. With my guidance and the guides' help, Jeff was able to identify and evict five very ominous entities. All were deeply entrenched, blocking his energy flow and impacting his physical body, causing him daily, chronic pain. With each being we removed, Jeff recalled a different surgery he had endured. It appeared that each of these entities had become embedded during one of his surgeries. Since he had been operated on many times, I asked whether he felt confident in his ability to repeat this process for himself. I explained that it was highly likely more entities would surface later. He assured me he was able and willing to do this for himself.

I outlined the shamanic journey process, and Jeff said he was ready to begin. He lay down and, once he was comfortable, I led him down the steps into the unconscious. I then directed him to call in a higher guide, which he did. Immediately, Jeff reported seeing a being before him but said the image was not very clear. He added that several other clouded forms came in with this guide. I instructed Jeff to ask the spirit its name, which I commonly do. The being replied, "I don't know my name. I am here with my friends." When Jeff relayed this response, I became slightly nauseous and suspicious of this spirit being and his friends. (Note: This particular session took place before I fully appreciated the crucial step of ascertaining the guide's purity of intent, and this experience convinced me of its importance.)

I told Jeff to ask this spirit if it was the right guide for the work we were to do. To this, the being answered, "Yes." I remained vigilant as I instructed Jeff to request that the spirit being take him to the originating cause of his obsession with cliffs. Within moments, Jeff reported that he was in a murky, unclear environment with "a larger gang of beings, in addition to the guide." Upon hearing his description of the shadowy domain and the gang, I became very concerned about our guide's integrity and the journey itself.

Jeff then said the beings all began talking to him at once, saying, "You are one of us. You are one with it all." I gave him a variety of questions to ask these spirits to glean some information about them. No matter what we asked them, they doggedly kept repeating the same words, like some kind of hypnotic chant. They would not explain who they were, nor what they meant by their repetitive words. This situation was unusual, and we were both displeased. It was clear we were not dealing with a genuine guide and that these spirit beings would be of no help.

I directed Jeff to ask the being if what was occurring here pertained to an oath Jeff had taken in a past life. The creature perked up and replied that it did. I decided not to ask about the oath or get more details because of my foreboding feelings. Gradually, a realization began to dawn on me that this event concerned a past life where Jeff had dabbled in alchemy and black magic. I felt we did not want to address the subject with this gang of spirits, and an alternate course of action arose. I directed Jeff to tell these beings that, in this present moment, he possessed complete and total free will. Moreover, he needed to inform them that he had the power, as a sovereign being, to declare that any oath taken in a past life was now null and void. He then decreed aloud, "I hereby dissolve and clear all oaths I have taken."

Jeff reported that the spirit beings became very angry at this action. They told him he couldn't get out of his oath, that it was unbreakable and binding. I counseled Jeff to reply, "So, you do not agree that, as a human being, I have complete and total free will?" They replied, "No, we do not recognize your free will." At this, I told Jeff to declare that since they did not honor his free will, they proved themselves spirits who were not in alignment with Divine Light and therefore were not welcome in his journey. I explained that they had to leave his presence and energy field immediately, at his command. He then cast them out with his decree, and they vanished like smoke. We were both relieved by their departure, and the murky environs of his journey space quickly cleared.

I asked Jeff to call for a new higher guide, and a light-filled being came in. We asked him three times if he was a being of the light, and he answered "yes" each time. I suggested Jeff ask this spirit being to help him with the past life where he had taken the oath mentioned by the nefarious beings. He did so, and was quickly transported to that past life. He saw that he had been a member of a community of sorcerers who were misusing their knowledge to try to gain power through alchemy. This revelation confirmed my earlier suspicions. Jeff told me how he had taken an eternal oath qualifying him to become a member of that community. Later, he had a change of heart and decided that he no longer wanted to be tied to them—but it was impossible to undo the binding oath. In his desperation, he killed himself by jumping off a high cliff.

The sinister beings of his community had somehow tracked Jeff into his current incarnation. Once they located him, they incessantly tried to influence him to jump off a cliff, thereby returning him to the spirit world where they could access him. I suggested that he ask if his spirit helper could clear the past-life energetic archive, the traumatic death and the oath. The guide assured him that he could, and I encouraged Jeff to formally request that all the secret agreements, oaths and energies of that lifetime be cleared and healed. Within seconds, the higher being told Jeff he had completed it. Next, I recommended that he ask his guide to fill the space where the oppressive energy had been with whatever Jeff chose to replace it. He asked to be filled with love, light and service to the Divine. Then he remarked that he could no longer feel his cliff obsession and instead was bathed with shining, ethereal energy.

The higher guide admonished Jeff to make more enlightened and empowered choices in the future, and Jeff promised to be more careful now that he understood their importance. The spirit being pledged that he would always be available for any further work that was needed. Jeff replied that he was very grateful for his guide's assistance, wisdom and counsel and that he would call upon him. I urged him to ask if there was a gift from Spirit that he could receive to use in his current lifetime. The shining guide replied, "Certainly," and proceeded to place several empowered talismans into Jeff's body while filling his aura with celestial light. He then counseled Jeff to remember that it is true that we are all one with All That Is. Jeff promised he would take that to heart.

I prompted Jeff to ask whether he needed any protection going forward in his life. The light being replied that love is Jeff's protection and that love is always there for him. This disclosure brought our journey to an end, and I asked Jeff to request that his guide return him to the gateway. Once there, he again expressed his gratitude to the spirit helper for the healing he had received and said he would be calling on the guide soon.

As I brought Jeff up the steps into our ordinary reality, he was beaming, filled to the brim with love and light. He was delighted to be back and remarked how free and unencumbered he felt. He told me that he had learned a great deal, especially about oaths, and knew that he would never again be obsessed with cliffs. I told him I was grateful that his issues had been revealed and cleared and encouraged him to continue working closely with his luminous guide. We then thanked our spiritual support team and closed sacred space.

* * *

Again, cleansings remove the outermost layer of coating energies—those that are in the auric field. The extraction of embodied stagnant energy addresses a second such stratum of energy deposits. We will explore more of these levels as we move along to further chapters. One of these layers contains *thought-forms* or *entities,* and I present this concept here since I have found these to be extremely common in clients.

Thought-forms are complexes of both mental and emotional energies generated by humans. We all commonly encounter these in daily life. Beliefs that we hold are one example of a thought-form. The ideas and beliefs instilled in us by parents, teachers, leaders or people we respect can be very powerful. From a shamanic perspective, thought-forms can become internalized over time and energized through constant reinforcement or feeding. With enough time, a thought-form can become a sentient creature. For example, a person consistently repeats internally, over many years, a judgment to which they were subjected. This energetic feeding of the thought-form produces what I refer to as an entity. I use the term *entity* as a practical tool for working with these complex energetic beings. The case study below highlights some examples of thought-forms that progressed into entities to give you a feel for the process.

* * *

Maria was referred to me by a long-time friend. When I first interviewed her, it was clear that she was a tremendously unhappy woman. For many years, she had been married to an alcoholic man who was in total denial about his condition. She asked me if I could help her resolve some of her marital issues. I replied that we could most likely get some clarity on her situation and proceed from there.

I greeted Maria at the door. She was a lovely Peruvian lady with beautiful long black hair. We entered my healing room, and I oriented her to my sacred altar. I told her that it was based upon ancestral Peruvian healing traditions, and she spent a few minutes admiring its complex configuration honoring the directions, elements and ancestors. Once she was seated and ready to begin the session, I asked her for more details about her relationship. She stated that her husband was an angry person who was resentful about his life. She further explained that he consistently projected his anger onto her, making her life a living hell. Not surprisingly, he had a mother who was also angry and never recognized anything good about her son. Maria was filled with sadness and despair about living in such a toxic environment but confided that she felt helpless to do anything about it. "He is a wealthy man," she said, and she had felt honored, years ago, that "such a rich and powerful man would even look at me." And this was the main reason she had married him.

Maria admitted that she had known about his problems and had minimized them, hoping he would change. She realized that she had done this all to herself and trapped herself for many years in a toxic marriage. I asked why she didn't leave him, and she replied that she did not believe she could make it on her own. She was convinced that she didn't have what it took to succeed. She had even created her own business in an attempt to support herself and gain independence. But the enterprise never did well, she explained, because her husband continually denigrated it and her, adding that he was always verbally and emotionally abusive to her. Maria had tried for many years to get him to stop drinking and incessantly watching TV to distract himself, but nothing had worked. She asked me again if I could help her.

I explained my understanding of the causes of addiction, why her husband behaved as he did, and what it would take for him to heal. I emphasized that he was the only one who could change himself. Maria assured me that she completely understood everything I said. I stressed that the only person she had any right, or potential, to change was herself, and she agreed that this was true. I added that, based on what she told me, the only hope I saw for her was to end her marriage. Although fearful of the thought of divorce, she now saw that trying to change him had not worked and never would. She acknowledged she had work to do and was willing to explore what lay beneath the surface.

Maria confided that she had no real friends in her life and added, "I do things, buy stuff and join clubs so that I will belong." These relationships were all shallow and empty, and she admitted that she had been "acting, trying to be liked and to belong," instead of being true to herself and doing what she wanted to do. "My family is not supportive," she told me. "They all live in Peru and do not really care about me."

I asked about her childhood, and Maria confided that she had been told repeatedly by her father that she was not good enough. She was the youngest child in her large family and broke so many things that her father told everyone in the family not to give her anything because she would break it. She was full of sadness and extensive programming, both from her husband and her father, and carried many unexamined wounds. I felt moved to help her look at them more closely.

Being from Peru, Maria was familiar with traditional forms of energy work, known as *curanderismo* in Spanish, and understood spiritual energies. I outlined the procedures I would use, and she agreed to participate. We began by opening sacred space and calling in our spiritual support. Conducting a series of energy cleansings using a Peruvian floral cologne, a feather fan and an empowered wooden staff, I removed considerable debris from her aura. She experienced the cleansings as having bands of heavy, dense energy peeled off, one by one, like the layers of an onion. I taught her how to do the cleansings and stressed that she would benefit from doing them regularly. She agreed to do them now that she understood their importance.

Next, I gave Maria a simple explanation of the types of acquired energies that can become embodied in a person. I told her I felt she had what I refer to as entities and explained about thought-forms. I used the "can't do anything right" energy that she was exposed to for her entire childhood as an example. Over many decades, this belief had become a conscious entity—a menacing, unpleasant creature that continually berated her. She understood exactly what I meant. I asked her to locate where it resided in her body, and she pointed to her solar plexus and said, "It is here." I told her to ask this creature its name, which she did. It would not respond, but as she asked it more questions, I could sense it. I asked Maria if she could perceive or communicate with it, and she replied that she could not. I then precisely explained my perceptions of it, and she acknowledged having the same feelings.

I asked Maria if she wanted to be rid of this being, to which she responded with a resounding "Yes!" I directed her to tell the energy in her solar plexus that it was an entity and not a part of her. At that point, it began to communicate with her, and she continued the expulsion, eventually calling in guides to permanently remove the creature. She reported that she felt much lighter once it was gone.

Maria and I proceeded with the process of discovering additional entities. Another one revealed itself to her, and she could easily communicate with it. This entity was also a self-sabotaging voice in her psyche that she recognized from childhood. It became more circumscribed as we worked with it, and she was finally able to enlist the guides to remove it.

Maria searched for more, and a third entity emerged. All her thoughts of being defective and not good enough appeared to have created this entity. As we addressed it, it stubbornly resisted the process and was unwilling to depart. I explained that this was common and guided her to call upon Archangel Michael to remove it. She reported that he appeared, completely removed the entity and took it away with him. She thanked Archangel Michael and said she was greatly relieved that this entity was gone.

Following that, I had Maria call upon the legendary Peruvian being named Naymlap. He is a spiritual ally with whom I work. She reported keenly feeling him as he came in to work with her. I directed her to request that he clear out all the toxic energetic debris accumulated in her body from the entities she had just removed, in alignment with her highest good. She stated this aloud and described her experience of him removing and clearing a considerable amount of shadowy, leaden energy from her body. I also felt the clearing in my body as it proceeded. When Naymlap finished, Maria thanked him, and he departed. I asked her how she was feeling, and she replied that she felt lighter, freer, more peaceful and much more spacious. We then called upon Archangel Michael to fill the spaces vacated by the entities with joy and peace. I complimented her on her ability to accomplish this intensive healing on herself.

Next, I gave Maria an overview of the shamanic journey, and she opted to lie down beside the altar for the process. I darkened the room, then led her into a deeply relaxed state and gradually walked her down into the unconscious, along a path, and through a gateway. I directed her to call in her higher guide. A shining being immediately appeared, and we ascertained that she was of the light and appropriate for the journey.

I suggested that Maria ask her luminous guide to show her the parameters around her disconnection from herself. She swiftly found herself observing a scene of her early childhood. She remembered being afraid of the dark and told me that she still feared many things. The spirit being explained that Maria was full of fear but had the power to release it. At that point, I handed her a 4-inch-long dark grey hematite extraction stone and explained that she could let all the fear she carried go into it. With great intent, she released her fear and reported feeling a huge discharge of energy from her body into the hematite. I directed her to ground this energy by blowing on the stone, sending the energetic contents into my altar.

The guide then expressed to Maria that she needed courage. I urged her to ask if the spirit helper would assist in filling her body with this attribute. The being readily agreed and, within moments, Maria excitedly told me she felt the energy of courage enter into every cell in her body. She began crying tears of joy as this new energy filled her. I felt the enormous impact this was having on her, and we paused for a few minutes to assimilate this powerful experience.

I then counseled Maria on the need to take responsibility for her own life. She agreed that there was nothing she could do for her husband and that she must save herself. She promised both her guide and me that she would take on this responsibility. The higher being told Maria to take time daily to pray, as prayer was her principal spiritual resource. She immediately consented to do this, and we conversed for a few minutes about the power of prayer. She shared that she was feeling much better—lighter, happier and more clearheaded.

The shining being then advised Maria that we had completed our work for the day. I directed her to ask to return to the gateway where the journey had begun, and she was instantly there. I reminded her to thank her higher being for all the healing she had received. The spirit helper assured Maria that she would always be available and would hear her every prayer.

When Maria was ready to return, I guided her up the steps, back into my healing room. She was smiling peacefully and looked physically lighter. We talked at length about her insights and feelings, and she slowly integrated her journey experiences. I then filled her aura with beneficial energies using floral waters, a feather and prayers, which gave her complexion a rosy cast. We concluded our session by thanking our spiritual support and closing sacred space.

Before leaving, Maria told me she would soon be going back to Peru for a full month. She would be visiting her family, she said, and was now feeling more confident that she could be her own person in their presence. I noticed she was standing much straighter as she spoke. I told her I believed she would be successful and wished her safe travels.

* * *

Anyone working in spiritual or shamanic circles knows that myriad spiritual beings inhabit the multiverse and that entities are among them. The term *entity* is hardly descriptive of such a varied class of beings; however, it is a commonly used term in shamanic and spiritual literature, and therefore is useful. The case study above has several examples of simple thought-form entities. This type of entity is usually connected to childhood programming by parents, teachers, society or peers and, like many other entities, tends to be denigrating, judgmental and punitive.

In my experience, many people carry conscious, disembodied, energetic beings that are not thought-forms. What these beings actually might be is unclear, as they appear to be a very diverse collection. What they all share is the trait of being conscious. When directly questioned, they will typically answer the person who addresses them. The entity's response might consist of a telepathic thought, a voice, movement in the body, pain, a knowing, or a feeling in the person housing the entity. These beings constitute a vast array of energetic types, from innocuous or even innocent to cunningly deceptive, malevolent or venomous. Sometimes the vile, malicious entities are connected to curses or black magic and can even be transmitted in family lineages.

All case studies presented in this book contain guided shamanic journeys. In other words, these are travels in consciousness into non-ordinary realities, including our personal and collective unconscious, and provide the opportunity to interact with a wide spectrum of spiritual beings. The main difference between the classic shamanic journey and the guided shamanic journeys I lead is that I actively guide the client in the journey to initiate direct contact with their spirit guide and request their own healing. This manner of working allows me to focus on the client's pertinent issues, move the journey process along and prevent the client from becoming stuck or lost in nonphysical realms.

I use this journey technique because it is a simple, direct and concise method to facilitate entry into other states of consciousness. Most people, though not all, can easily do this imaginal traveling. The individual enters a very light trance state and, due to the enhanced level of suggestibility involved, every practitioner must maintain the highest ethical behavior. There are a great many books on shamanism and shamanic journeying for the reader to explore.

Chapter 5

Basic Guidelines and Extraction Process

WHAT SKILLS AND QUALITIES SHOULD a facilitator have to offer these healing techniques? Deep compassion and love are essential, along with a genuine interest in the spiritual realms and how those realms interact with us. It is beneficial to have a working relationship with spiritual guides, animal allies, totems, ancestors or higher-density light beings. It is also desirable to have experience or training in energy healing, psychology, bodywork, shamanism, alchemy, qi gong, metaphysics, sacred plant medicine, or any healing art. Direct personal experience of Spirit, mystical states, non-ordinary or quantum realities gives the practitioner flexibility, depth and creativity. The qualities of patience, focused intention, high integrity and a non-judgmental attitude are prerequisites for any healing practice.

The facilitator must hold the sacred container for the work, as it is the energetic expanse in which all healing takes place. Utilizing a sacred altar of any kind facilitates the creation and maintenance of the container and sacred space. It also serves as a focal point for contact and communication with the spirit realm. Thus, it should be of the highest vibration and treated with great respect. Many sacred altars I have used descend from traditional Peruvian *mesa* lineages. A mesa is an ancient form of sacred altar created, activated and empowered using shamanic wisdom and generating deep transformative power. Ultimately, the desire to be of selfless service to others in a healing capacity is the motivation for doing this work, and your experience and spirit guides will be the best teachers.

Employing a protocol ensuring that only beings of light enter the healing space is another necessary aspect. I try not to use the terms *good* and *evil*, as they are value judgments, and instead use the words *light* and *dark* as more neutral observations to distinguish between energies, intentions and outcomes. In general, beings of light are expansive and promote growth, wholeness and healing, whereas beings of darkness are contractive and promote constriction and fragmentation. My guides have strongly emphasized the importance of working only with expansive light beings to ensure optimal health-giving results.

In a larger sense, we know the dark is part of the light, and what we perceive as darkness is something that has separated from the light and forgotten what it is. Shadowy beings are drawn toward the light but do not know how to enter into it. Instead, they seek to pull people who carry considerable light but are unwary into the dark vibrations because they want the energy of that light for themselves. These murky beings can be very persuasive, impressive, influential and seemingly have impressive powers and credible advice. They can also be deceptive, untruthful, parasitic and controlling, even promising to perform amazing feats for you.

In my experience, all ominous beings will demand payment for the actions they have taken or the information they've provided, which can create unnecessary problems. The principal manner of discerning the dark intentions from the light is through their communication and actions and your feelings. Beings who are of the light will be respectful, uplifting, loving, supportive, inclusive, compassionate and truthful. Light beings never ask for a payment, as they are in the service of love, healing, abundance and compassion. They may occasionally ask one to perform specific actions or make offerings in some manner; however, these are not payments per se but requests that address the balancing of all the energies involved on a larger scale.

The client's active participation in these healing modalities is essential. I recommend inviting people to assist you in creating the sacred container and calling in spirit guides as a potent way to begin your healing sessions. In addition to being inclusive, it allows the practitioner to ascertain a person's level of sensitivity to nonphysical energy and their willingness to engage in the process. Ideally, the individual coming for healing will also have some familiarity with the energetic universe and nonphysical realities; however, their desire to heal and their openness to exploring potentially challenging emotions and experiences are the key traits. The client must be motivated and have the capacity to be guided into altered states of consciousness and interact with spirit beings. In other words, the person must be willing to face their own shadow and the unknown. It is paramount for the individual to have considerable trust in the person facilitating these processes.

* * *

Marisol was a vivacious young woman with a huge heart. She was a previous student who had recently been through a series of grueling health challenges and was still struggling with them. She asked for my help, explaining that she wanted to end her attachment to "the pain experience." She told me she experienced significant daily pain and was concerned that she would always be in pain. Also, she said that her ancestors "were feeding off of my energy" and that she had unhealthy connections to them. We agreed to do a healing session to see what we could uncover.

I was happy to see Marisol again and gave her a long hug. Once she was oriented to my healing room, we opened sacred space and engaged our spiritual support. I began with basic energy cleansings and found that she had many layers of obstructing energy that I pulled from her aura and discharged into my altar ground. I strongly recommended performing these cleansings daily to keep the debris from accumulating and disrupting her energy bodies. We reviewed the techniques for enacting the cleansings until she was comfortable with them and committed to doing them daily.

I seated Marisol in front of my altar, and she spent several minutes connecting with the many crystals on it. I pointed out my favorite extraction stone and told her its name. I then explained how to use it to remove the internalized heavy energy in her body. As we talked, she said she could already feel a lot of thick, tarry energy in her body. She picked up the large tourmaline from the altar and energetically connected to it. I slowly walked her through the extraction process and then let her proceed. After a few minutes, she reported that considerable noxious energy had come into her right shoulder, as she intended it to, and then exited her body, flowing into the stone. She said she felt the stone helping her by pulling on the energies that needed to be released. When she finished the extraction, I gave her another stone from my altar to carry out extractions at home and explained how to care for it.

Next, we moved on to a discussion of the entities I knew she was carrying. After a general description of these energy beings, I began helping her find those residing in her body by asking her a series of questions about her feelings and perceptions. She had no trouble identifying several ominous and hostile entities that were causing some of her physical pain. She expelled these beings as she focused on them and followed my guidance for their removal. She told me she had recently been hospitalized several times and was sure that she had acquired these entities there. I replied that many people I have worked with recounted similar stories.

I then prepared her for the shamanic journey, giving her an overview of the procedure. I darkened the room as she lay on a pad beside the altar. When she was relaxed and comfortable, I led her down the steps into the unconscious and directed her to call in a higher guide. Mary Magdalene immediately appeared to her, and she remarked that she had lately worked closely with her as a guide. Mary confirmed that she was of the light, so I instructed Marisol to ask to see all the details around her seemingly endless pain. She reported being shown an image of herself holding down the corner of a large woven blanket, which represented the healing of her ancestral lineages. Mary explained that Marisol's pain was attached to this lineage healing issue but that these ancestral matters did not relate to or depend upon Marisol personally.

"You do not have to hold the blanket," Mary said to her. Marisol admitted that she strongly felt this healing task was necessary and that it fell to her as the best person in her family to accomplish it. I urged her to inquire about the conditions lying behind this situation. Mary explained a broad lineage agreement existed, stipulating that a living descendant would serve as an energy source for the family's ancestors. This agreement explained the chronic energy drain. Marisol then realized that she had accepted the responsibility for this ancestral healing because of her high sensitivity to subtle energies, especially those of her lineage. She stated that this had now become her life commitment to her ancestors. Mary explained that these ancestors were hungry and desperate for many reasons, which was why they continually pulled life-force energy from her.

I urged Marisol to ask what options existed—what she could do to address her agreement. Mary's recommendation was for her to "study some form of martial art to develop a warrior mindset." She then added that Marisol must use the discipline of the martial art to hone her sense of herself until she could see and work with the ancestral agreement to which she had committed herself. I asked Marisol if all of this made sense to her, and she replied that she had been getting the martial arts message for several months but didn't know what it meant because there was no context. Now that she understood the push to learn a martial art, she stated she was ready to undertake it.

As soon as Marisol voiced her new resolve, another spirit being—who was carrying an elaborate, long sword—appeared. This guide approached, presented the carved sword to Marisol, and instructed her to begin practicing her martial art training with this sword, in non-ordinary reality, every day. Before departing, the being also revealed that a physical sword would soon be coming into her life, after which she should continue the training with the new sword. We were both very intrigued by this event and wondered what could be next.

Mary Magdalene continued by telling Marisol she was to build an ancestor shrine. This shrine had to be an actual, physical altar created in whatever way she chose. When she completed the altar, Mary explained, she must then make a doll and transfer all of her pain into it. "The doll will take the pain," Mary said, adding that Marisol must then place the doll on the ancestor shrine and leave it there. Mary continued speaking for a few minutes, giving Marisol more detailed instructions about her tasks and how to fulfill them. I asked her if she felt she would be able to complete this assignment, and she replied with confidence, "Yes, I can."

Mary had also instructed Marisol to have better boundaries, meaning not to let her ancestors attach to her at will. Marisol found it difficult to imagine having better boundaries but understood their impact since she was now beginning to see her enmeshment with all the ancestor energies. Mary then provided her with a detailed explanation of the importance of good boundaries and insisted that she make a verbal agreement to create and maintain them.

When Marisol finished making her pledge, Mary gave her yet another assignment: to commit to doing some form of creative expression every day. Marisol, she said, was to engage and utilize her creative energies in whatever manner she chose, as long as it was sincere. Marisol agreed to this, and Mary also requested her to affirm it aloud.

I suggested that Marisol ask if she had any fragments we could retrieve during this journey, which she promptly did. Within moments, she reported being in a place where she could see four soul pieces and knew that each was connected to one of her four grandparents. Mary explained that these fragments also represented her four ancestral lineages through her grandparents. I told her to ask Mary to facilitate returning each of these fragments into her body, which she quickly completed. Mary then revealed that the ability of that particular lineage to negatively impact Marisol diminished as each fragment was reintegrated. We were both pleased to hear this good news.

Next, Mary explained that each of Marisol's four lineages contained considerable black magic and curses and detailed how these functioned.

Marisol vowed that she was committed to clearing these curses in future work, and I replied that I would be happy to help her with this endeavor.

I then prompted Marisol to ask if there was any past-life trauma that we could heal. Mary replied that there was, but we had done enough for one day, and the past-life issues would have to wait for another session. I asked Marisol to request that Mary return her to the gateway, and she said she was there. I reminded her to thank Mary Magdalene for all the healing and wisdom she had provided. Marisol did this immediately and told Mary she would be calling on her again soon.

When Marisol was ready, I guided her up the steps into our everyday world. I opened the curtains as she was sitting up, and we chatted about the journey and her extensive assignments. She was happy to have received such clear information about the ancestral issues and reaffirmed her determination to follow through with all her tasks, "no matter what." I asked how she was feeling, and she said she felt considerably better and that her pain had diminished some from the work we had done. I told her she looked much less stressed than she had before the session. I then filled her aura with prayers and light using rose water and a feather to sustain her for the work ahead, and then ensured that she was grounded. She thanked me for my guidance, saying she would like to do another session soon. I replied that I would be happy to work with her whenever she was ready. We then closed sacred space, thanking our spirit helpers for their service.

Shortly after this session, Marisol moved out of state. She stays in touch and has continued to work on healing her lineage, clearing the curses and black magic and healing herself. She has since decided to go back to school to earn a professional degree and recently became engaged.

* * *

Stone Extraction Process
Overview:

In the case studies presented, I frequently employ a stone to extract dense energies that can cause blocks within a client's body. These energies are inside the body rather than in the aura and must be drawn out or expelled. Extractions take place within the context of a healing session where sacred space has been opened and a good container has been created for this work. There are many methods of using a stone to remove subtle energies from the body. I typically use the following process since it is uncomplicated and easy to follow.

First, acquaint yourself with a suitable stone. Ideally, it will be about fist-sized—also dark, heavy and dense, like the energies you want it to extract. Meteorites, hematite, obsidian and black basalt are examples of ideal stones. Next, ask the stone if it is willing to be of service as your extraction stone. If the stone agrees, you can use it. If it says no, do not use it and seek another one. Once you have your stone, you need to cleanse it of any previous programming, using your favored smoke, water or sound and your intention to remove this energy.

Ask the stone if it has a name, and use that name to call it into service each time you employ it. If it does not, the two of you can choose a name you both would like to use. You must <u>inform</u> the stone of the service you want it to provide, which becomes a program held in the stone. In this case, tell the stone you want it to be your extraction stone to pull dense, heavy, stagnant and obstructing energies from the people who hold it. You can then empower your stone by rubbing it with sweet-smelling waters (such as rose) or passing it through uplifting smoke (such as copal). If you have an altar, the stone should rest there when not in use. If you do not have an altar, keep your stone in a sacred place, preferably in your healing room.

Exclusively use your right hand to pick up and hold the stone whenever you use it to extract energy. We do this because energy enters the body via the left hand and passes from the body via the right. Thus, since you will be removing undesirable energy, you use only your right hand. You do not need to access the story or content held in these frequencies, since it is best to relate to them purely energetically. Some people worry about contaminating the Earth with these heavy energies. Native wisdom teaches us that this is never a problem because the Earth receives and transmutes them—just like compost—and puts them back where they belong.

Step-by-step process:

1. Pick up the stone with your right hand and say the stone's name aloud to engage it. Remind it that you would like it to help you extract heavy, dense, obstructing energies.

2. As you take in a normal breath, intend, will, imagine, command or decree that all blocking energies come from wherever they are in your body and gather in your right shoulder.

3. As you breathe out, send these energies down your right arm and into the stone. You may feel the stone getting heavy or cold, or feel it pulling the energies out of you as you do this.

4. Continue doing this procedure, using your normal breath, until you feel the process has finished—this usually only takes a few minutes.

5. Once you have accomplished the extraction, discharge the collected energies by blowing them from the stone into the ground (if indoors, this will be the floor). Remember, it is your intention to discharge the energies that achieves this.

6. Cleanse your stone with smoke (such as sage) or waters (like rue), thank the stone for its service, and replace it on your altar using your right hand.

If you are guiding someone in this work, you direct the person to follow the steps above, walking them through each part of the process. For this technique, the client must perform the extraction on themselves. You will guide and assist them in the process, answer questions and hold space. The extraction can be a very subtle experience; however, most people will perceive that something has happened and many will distinctly feel the energy leaving their body and accumulating in the stone. Again, it is crucial to discharge the collected energy into the ground and to cleanse your stone to complete the process.

Chapter 6

A Perspective on Energy Healing

Energy healing relies on both physical and nonphysical sources. Although neglected by science for centuries, the nonphysical sources are crucial in healing much chronic dis-ease. Many energy healers, as well as other practitioners, view a large portion of illness—especially chronic conditions—as arising from unresolved emotional trauma. This suffering is deposited energetically in our physical and nonphysical bodies. It does not dissipate or go away by itself but stays there until it is released or transmuted. The first law of thermodynamics states that heat energy can neither be created nor destroyed; heat energy can only be transferred or changed from one form to another. I believe this law also applies to spiritual forms of energy and is essentially how much energy healing works. I am not referring to acute or infectious diseases here, although I believe that most illnesses have multiple causes, among which are energetic conditions.

The potential sources of trauma in humans are vast, yet much of what I encounter in my healing practice is unresolved archived trauma from a person's current lifetime. Most commonly, the distress occurred in early childhood or even in utero, although it can originate in any stage of one's life. Sometimes the trauma has caused fragments of an individual to split off, in what is referred to in shamanism as *soul loss*. The condition is healed by locating the missing pieces and returning it in a process called *soul retrieval*.

The topic of past lives comes up frequently in my work, and whatever past lives are, they seem to be a source of considerable unresolved trauma. The affliction is typically connected to the death of the person or a loved one in a particular past life, but it can also be an incarnational theme that spans several past lives. Many of the case studies presented in this book describe journeys into past lives to clear archived trauma. The concept of past lives forms a convenient and useful model through which much healing can occur, and whether or not one believes in past lives makes no difference. Our mainstream culture's denial of past lives, reincarnation and the survival of consciousness after death does not appear to influence an individual's journey experience.

The key for both practitioner and client is to have an open mind when approaching spiritual energy healing. If a person can entertain the concept long enough to have a direct experience of being taken to view a past life, their personal experience will be deeply healing. Considerable emotion may arise during one's encounter with a past life, providing the opportunity to feel and release embedded emotions, which is inherently cathartic. I have never had a client question their direct experiences of the journey; most report having a knowing, beyond a shadow of a doubt, that they did experience themselves in that lifetime. In other words, past lives are real and self-evident to the journeyer. Occasionally, additional memories of that life will continue to return to the individual's conscious awareness in response to visiting it.

Martha's story illustrates the power of archived emotions from a past life. The specific issue she wanted to address was the deep feeling of sadness she had experienced for her entire life, more than four decades. During her shamanic journey, when we asked her guide to take her to the source of her enduring sadness, she immediately found herself in a past life. She recounted the scene to me in great detail as she viewed it. Martha observed herself as a five-year-old girl, standing alone in a hayfield. She was watching as her family's beautiful white farmhouse and two-story barn burned to the ground. She agitatedly reported that her entire family was trapped in the house, and she knew that all of them had died. Martha described seeing the fiercely blazing barn and hearing the screaming horses penned inside as they burned alive. The full impact of this event washed over her as she narrated it to me, and she began to sob and wail. It was heart-rending to witness her vividly re-experiencing the loss of everything she knew.

Martha's crying continued in waves for many minutes as each new realization broke on the shore of her consciousness. Her mother, father, brother and sister, her favorite horse, all the animals—everything in her life was gone. From my perception, she allowed the entire archive of her horror and grief to come through her, be deeply felt, and then released. After quite a while, the emotional process ran its course, and she began to talk about all her feelings and experience surrounding the tragedy. We integrated this archive into her current life as more and more insights arose for her. Martha underwent an immense transformation through her willingness to experience her past-life despair.

I have occasionally heard healing professionals say it is not beneficial to re-traumatize people by having them face a disturbing event from their past. Maybe this does not apply to past-life events, or perhaps one's guides will censor the event if it is too traumatic. My impression of Martha was that it was her choice to experience, process and release the archived trauma and that her emotional re-encounter was paramount to the healing she derived from it. It is possible that being in an altered state during the shamanic journey may reduce the likelihood of re-traumatization since this has also been observed with psychedelic-assisted therapy.

Another common source of archived trauma can be one's ancestors. In these cases, the original trauma belonged to someone in the ancestral lineage, either a direct ancestor or a family member of an ancestor. The initial emotional trauma, for whatever reason, was suppressed and unresolved, and this censoring caused the trauma energy to embed in the body of that person. We now know that our emotions interact with our neuro-immuno-endocrine system to produce physical tags, known as epigenetic markers, on our DNA. Epigenetic markers control gene expression and represent a direct physical mechanism for transmitting emotional trauma, and the diseases that these can cause, to future generations.

Epigenetic research reveals that emotional distress can create changes to molecules in the body and that these changes can subsequently be inherited for multiple generations. The science of epigenetics has become an exciting field of study as we discover more of these mechanisms. I encourage anyone interested in these topics to research this emerging field.

It has been my experience that nonphysical modes of transmission exist in the energy bodies, especially the emotional body. Somehow, emotional pain from a past life is transmitted to a current one, leaving a discoverable energetic imprint. Is this transmission spiritual? Could this be how karma works? How spiritual transmission might occur is a mystery; however, quantum potential—a sub-quantum field comprised of information—could be one mechanism for it.

A further category of damage, one that we all share, is collective or transpersonal trauma. Our history is replete with examples, including many millennia of conquest, genocide, wars, massacres, ethnic cleansing, the Holocaust, racism, sexism, and the spiritual trauma of the desecration of the Divine Feminine. These wounds are rooted in each of us—from ancient times to the present—and remain unresolved in the collective human psyche. We are now beginning to witness the surfacing and resolution of some of our transpersonal trauma on the world stage.

At this time, there is a widespread awakening of humanity to the ancient understanding that we are all related and interconnected, and this is Unity Consciousness. Theoretical physicist Dr. David Bohm referred to this as *wholeness* and understood that all existence is fundamentally connected as consciousness or information in a multidimensional reality. This description is also what the world's mystics tell us, but it has yet to be accepted by our modern science other than quantum mechanics. I believe we are slowly coming to realize that we have been living in a spiritually underdeveloped culture.

As we awaken to the direct gnosis that we are all inextricably joined in the web of life, more and more people will understand the necessity of resolving our collective trauma—as it is unquestionably impeding our species' evolution of consciousness. Much exciting healing work is now occurring in the field of collective trauma psychology. Furthermore, I trust that our nascent awakening into Unity Consciousness will heal the sources of our collective trauma, part of which is the delusion that anything is separate from everything else. Unity Consciousness means it will be self-evident to everyone that there is no separation between people, between humans and the rest of creation, or within creation itself, be it physical or energetic.

We know that trapped energy blocks normal biological processes, which may then cause dysfunction in healthy systems, and can even promote adaptive responses that may turn out to be unhealthy. Energy medicine and energy psychology are fascinating fast-emerging fields of healing practice employing this knowledge. For example, *Thought Field Therapy* has now become an evidence-based treatment for trauma and stress disorders.

Research has demonstrated that archived energies can be impacted by the frequencies of sound, Reiki and even pure consciousness itself. We know that intention can change reality at the quantum level. In 1931, physicist Max Planck wrote: "I regard consciousness as fundamental. I regard matter as derivative from consciousness."[5] It is now undeniable that consciousness continuously impacts us via energetic and spiritual realities. Therefore, it is time to enlist these in the service of healing on a larger scale.

I have long envisioned embedded trauma in the form of "packets" of archived energy that can reside in both physical and nonphysical realities. These packets, sequestered in our corporeal and energetic bodies, can be the source of dis-ease, can be transmitted to descendants, and can even be passed on to future selves in future lifetimes. Since this archived energy is readily accessed spiritually, my focus has been to address and heal it using spiritual means.

This approach is not the only way to transform archived energy, as many other energy healing techniques are also effective. We know that all energy affects us and can initiate myriad diseases that impact the physical, mental, emotional and spiritual bodies. That recent research supports an energetic etiology for depression, anxiety, PTSD, OCD, addiction, phobias, stress-related illness, autoimmune disorders, mental illness and cancers is reason enough to expand energy healing technologies throughout our healthcare system. I have not had clients with serious mental illness and have not seen research on using energy healing modalities with this cohort. However, I think this could be a valuable area of future study.

I continue to be impressed that we can directly address a great deal of illness using spiritual methods. The healing techniques presented in this book do not require any particular spiritual belief or level of attainment. Using very simple progressive relaxation or hypnosis-type induction, a practitioner can guide a client into an altered state and enlist spiritual helpers to convey the individual to the inception of their dis-ease. Assisted by wise higher beings, we can actively experience the energetic contents of archived trauma packets. Understanding the etiology of the dis-ease facilitates healing, and we can request that the guides transform the archived energy, thereby clearing the condition.

The investigation of spirituality and consciousness as an emerging approach to healing deserves serious research. Whether trauma packets are inherited physically, emotionally, spiritually, or all the above does not matter. Higher guides have the wisdom and capacity to clear and heal archived energy and to repair any damage the trauma may have caused. Further, there appear to be appropriate spirit guides who are ever willing to facilitate our requested healing. In other words, these light beings can clear, heal and resolve illness and trauma, and they will generally do so if asked by the individual who seeks their help. In the few exceptions to this that I have seen, the guides have made it clear that the request is ultimately not in a person's best interest or that the trauma serves an educational purpose for that individual's current incarnation.

A bonus for those benefiting from this type of energy healing is that it restores spiritual health and connection, vital to our overall health and well-being. Good spiritual health involves having faith, trust and a relationship with the Divine, Great Spirit, Source, Creator, or the Universe. Many clients have expressed their joy and gratitude in being connected, or reconnected, to their spirit guides. This connection in itself is incredibly healing and validating for the person and allows them to continue consciously working with their higher guide.

* * *

Julie, a healing professional and friend of many years, had worked with me sporadically in the past. This time she contacted me to help her with her intractable feelings of low self-worth and problems with charging money for her services. Being self-employed, both of these represented significant blocks. I interviewed her to gather additional information about her parents, her childhood and her belief systems. She had suffered considerable physical and emotional abuse throughout her childhood, which strongly affected her current sense of herself. I encouraged her to come in for a session with a guided shamanic journey.

Julie was of medium build with light brown hair and dressed in a lovely, flowing teal blouse. It was always a delight to work with her, I thought, as we walked into my healing room. Standing next to the altar, we opened our sacred space and called in spiritual support. I embarked on the series of energy cleansings, removing several congested layers from her aura. I then reminded her that she needed to take responsibility for doing regular cleansings at home.

Following that, I asked her to sit on a large zafu in front of my altar. She noticed I had a new sable obsidian sphere, and I told her that I had purchased it in Mexico several months previously. I discussed extractions and guided her to use the black tourmaline to extract additional troublesome energy from her physical body. When she finished the extraction process, she remarked that she already felt much lighter and would add extractions to her routine, too.

We moved on to address the entities I sensed Julie was carrying, and she located several that, with the guide's help, were not difficult for her to evict. One of these was a curious entity that I labeled "a deceiver." It was a shape-shifter and proceeded to morph into different forms and move around in her body as we tried to pin it down. It emitted what I perceived as a frequency or force, pushing me to look away and not see it. I have occasionally encountered entities that appear to broadcast energy, thoughts or influence, as this one did, which I find fascinating. However, I did not look the other way, nor did Julie as she engaged the guides to take it away to its proper realm.

I then reviewed the guided shamanic journey format, and Julie chose to remain sitting for the process. She possessed the rare ability to journey within the multiverse at will. I asked her to go into the unconscious, and Julie said she was already there and calling in her higher guide. She promptly announced that Mother Mary had come in to guide her. We posed some questions to be sure it was Mother Mary since malign beings can be convincingly deceptive.

Next, I suggested she ask Mary to bring her birth father, who was deceased, into her presence since he was the source of some of the abuse she had suffered as a young child. Julie made the request and stated that he suddenly appeared before her in his etheric body. I encouraged her to take this opportunity to tell him everything she felt about him as her father.

This process was deeply emotional for Julie, and it took her quite a while, with many tears, to say it all. When she finished, I directed her to tell her father that he could now say whatever he wanted her to know. He began speaking, and Julie was quite surprised by both his words and his tone of voice. He was no longer the conflicted, angry person he had been and had only loving, consoling and healing words for her. They conversed for many minutes, covering a wide range of topics, and then she stated that they had amicably resolved some of the issues they had had with each other when he had been alive.

I encouraged her to tell him all her thoughts and emotions so that she could finally resolve them. When she felt satisfied with her encounter, she said goodbye and asked Mary to take her father back to where he belonged. Julie was still teary-eyed and emotional but said she was feeling a great sense of relief. I congratulated her on her courage to face her father and work through so much intense material.

Next, I directed Julie to ask Mary to bring in her stepfather. Like her father, he was no longer incarnated and had also been physically and emotionally abusive to her. Mary immediately brought him before her, and I encouraged Julie to tell him how she felt about him, which she did. When she finished, we gave him his turn to speak. Julie sadly reported that, with forceful words and a harsh tone of voice, he told her that all the abuse and mean-spirited things he had done to her as a child had been good for her. He justified his harmful behavior by saying it had taught her a lot about life and, therefore, the abuse had actually benefited her.

I asked Julie how she felt about her stepfather's words, and she replied that it made her feel miserable and even caused her to doubt herself and the things she had told him. I noted that she automatically accepted his statements as the truth and found fault with herself. I explained that his words felt like pure rationalization to me, and even though he was in the astral plane, his behavior was the same as it had been when he was in physical form. "He's being a bully and is still stuck in his personal material," I offered. Julie and I discussed his defensiveness—that instead of doing his inner work, he blamed her. She said this had been his exact behavior toward her when she was a child.

Julie thought about it and agreed that he was not taking any responsibility for what he had done. With genuine sadness, she saw he had not changed at all. I explained my understanding of the astral plane and how no one is ever forced into realizations; everyone sees what they are ready to see. It became clear to Julie that she could not resolve anything with her stepfather until he progressed further in his evolution. I concurred, adding that he might not be ready for a long time, and urged her to address the energy he had directed toward her. I suggested that her guide might be able to remove all projections that had ever come from her stepfather and return that same energy to him. She requested this, and Mary replied, "I shall do it." Both of us had the sensation of thick, toxic energy lifting off Julie and depositing on her stepfather.

Julie then realized that she wanted to separate herself from her stepfather's influence and requested that Mary facilitate this for her. Mary fulfilled her request in an instant. When I asked her how she felt, she replied, "I feel free, completely separated from his domination, and clean in a way I have not felt in many years." She then asked Mary to take her stepfather back into the ethers, and he disappeared. We paused for a few minutes to give her time to enjoy her new good feelings and to let them assimilate.

Next, I suggested Julie ask her guide to take her to the inception of her money issues. She suddenly found herself in a past life where she saw that she was a sorcerer who took money from people to perform black magic and cast spells. Julie told me she caused harm to many people and took everyone's money even if her spells did not work. She could see a great cloud of dreadful energy surrounding that lifetime and the shadow that those actions cast on her current life. I guided her to ask if Mary could clear this grim, shadowy energy from both past and present lifetimes. Mary's answer was, "Of course," and Julie requested that she remove it at once.

Mary then brought forth several other past incarnations for Julie to witness, all of which carried the same basic theme as the first one. She again requested healing for these damaging and sinister energies, and Mary proceeded to clear them all. As this was happening, Julie exclaimed that she had experienced an intense energetic sensation, as if a substantial internal shift had occurred in her body, and that she now felt much more balanced.

I prompted Julie to ask if these past lives were responsible for her disinterest in genuinely caring for herself, and Mary replied that this was indeed the case. Julie acknowledged that self-care had always been a big challenge and asked Mary to help her begin some new good habits. Mary assured her that she is always with her and will help her whenever she asks. I encouraged Julie to make her new self-care habits more tangible by making a verbal pledge to Mary and me to be responsible for herself, first and foremost. Startled, she questioned me, saying, "Before my sons and before my clients and everyone else?" I replied, "Yes, before all of them." She told me she could not make that pledge because it would be too difficult for her to keep.

We then embarked on a discussion about Julie's responsibility to care for her physical body while on this planet. I explained that she freely chose this incarnation, that it was uniquely hers, and that she alone was responsible for herself. "It's like they say on the airplane," I added. "You have to put your oxygen mask on first before trying to help others." To play the game of life, you have to have a biological body, and every adult has the responsibility to maintain that body to stay on the physical plane. She thought about this for a few minutes, finally agreed it made sense to her and said she was willing to change.

I asked Julie again if she would like to pledge that she would do her best to take responsibility for herself first, and she replied that she could now make it. As she declared her vow aloud, we both felt an immense energetic alignment happening in her body and energy field—that is, I felt the alignment in my body as it happened to her. She excitedly told me that "as the alignment clicked in, [she] felt an immense flow of new energy coming into [her] body and mind." She interpreted this inflow as a powerful spiritual blessing, and these sublime feelings persisted for many minutes.

Julie had received a significant download, and I explained that it might take a while for her to integrate it completely. I recommended that she be very patient and observe the changes in her self-care habits as they unfolded, assuring her they would come. I told her this new energy would function as a template or blueprint to develop healthy habits and suggested devoting time and energy to manifest them in her daily life. Julie replied that she had just received the same information from Mary and vowed to remember it. We both had to laugh at that.

Mary then told us we had done enough work for one session, and I directed Julie to go back to her starting point for the journey. Once there, she thanked Mother Mary for all the healing work and promised to call on her again soon. When Julie was ready, I asked her to come back into our consensual reality, which she promptly did.

As Julie adjusted to the late afternoon light in the room, I noticed that she now looked quite different than she had when we started our session.

She had more vibrancy and animating life-force energy about her, her face looked more vital and healthy, and she was smiling. When I asked how she felt, she replied that she was exceptionally clear-headed and very grateful. Most exciting was the profound shift she could feel in her body and consciousness, and she expressed her total surprise that something like that could even happen. I replied that I shared her feelings—that it was miraculous to witness—and I was pleased that she had received such significant healing.

I asked Julie what her plans were for implementing a new self-care regimen. She promised me this would now be a top priority and thanked me for moving her onto a new path. I told her she was welcome and assured her that she could call on Mary and me if she got stuck or needed help making changes. After chatting for a while longer, we expressed our gratitude to our spirit helpers and closed sacred space.

About a month later, Julie called to tell me how much she had changed. She excitedly reported that she felt like she was a new human being. The old issues that had always stopped her in her tracks were now undetectable. It was much easier to make good choices, she added, and those choices just seemed to come naturally. Julie thanked me again for my guidance and the healing she had received, and I replied that I was elated for her.

Chapter 7

Ancestor Healing

ANCESTRAL CONTACT HAS BEEN PRACTICED since time immemorial, but we, in modern Western culture, have forgotten both how to contact ancestors and why it is valuable to do so. Who are our ancestors? We usually know our immediate forebears. However, our human ancestors go back eons—200,000 years or more—in an unbroken chain to Africa. In the larger sense, our ancestors are all humans who have lived before us, especially if they have left a legacy that impacts our lives in the present. Most of the healing work I do focuses on ancestors who have died in the recent historical past, as these ancestors have the most influence over us in the present. The vast majority of people on the planet believe that consciousness survives the death of the body and that we all enter some form of an afterlife. Thus, most people understand that when you die, you do not cease to exist.

The idea that our ancestors might need healing is new and possibly confusing to many people in Western culture; nevertheless, ancestor healing is slowly reappearing as a valuable and powerful practice. Why would our ancestors need healing? Which ancestors might need it? These are good questions, as not all ancestors require healing. Most are *healthy* or *well* ancestors, while others are entangled to some extent in experiences or conditions that they have not yet resolved.

Dr. Daniel Foor's important book *Ancestral Medicine: Rituals for Personal and Family Healing* has increased my understanding and given me a greater context for the healing work I do. His book also contains guided shamanic journeys that can address and resolve numerous ancestor issues, along with a wealth of information.

In my work, I have encountered five classes of ancestors who might need our help. These five are:

1. Recent ancestors from whom we have inherited unexamined emotional trauma

2. Unwell ancestors from one's lineage whose trauma has kept them trapped

3. Our collective ancestors who have been forgotten by present generations

4. Ancestors of the land who are long forgotten, including ancient ones whose bones are interred on their traditional land, giving them a deep connection to it

5. The troubled dead and ghosts who are still attached to the physical plane

We can enlist the higher guides to address ancestral and intergenerational trauma and other dysfunctional family patterns. Much healing can occur for both parties when a living person assists those who have died to complete their transition to the next phase of existence. The research on the epigenetics of trauma and the understanding of how it can be inherited can motivate us to heal those from whom we inherited unresolved emotional baggage. I have not seen this aspect of ancestor healing discussed in trauma research, but I think it should be.

Mark Wolynn's book, *It Didn't Start With You* is an excellent resource for understanding inherited trauma and the resulting problems spawned by it. He also provides potent exercises for healing intergenerational trauma, which function on emotional, mental and physical levels. His book does not discuss the healing of one's ancestors, but it can help you identify an ancestor who needs healing assistance. In other words, when you discover the person from whom you inherited an energetic charge, you then have the option to help them clear and resolve the trauma that your ancestor still carries. The case study below illustrates ancestral healing within the shamanic journey process.

* * *

My dear friend Emma called one day to ask if I could help her uncover what lay beneath a feeling she had lived with her entire life. The feeling was not always present but arose, persisted for months or years, and then submerged again into her unconscious. I asked her to tell me more, and she replied that it was the feeling she should kill herself. This suicidal urge manifested as a feeling of despair that painted life as tragic and continuing to worsen. At these times, she felt like there was no way out and that suicide was the only answer. Emma disclosed that she had often envisioned how she would end her life but had not acted upon those thoughts. I told her I felt I could help her find answers to this long-standing issue.

Emma, a senior who looked much younger than her age, arrived in jeans and a Hawaiian tank top. We hugged, and then I ushered her into my healing room. She admired the photos of saints and teachers on my altar, asking me who each one was. As she settled in, I asked her to assist me in opening sacred space and calling in our spiritual support. She commented that she felt the energy in the room shift as we did that and was looking forward to our session. I outlined the nature of the work, how it would proceed, and the importance of her participation, to which she cheerfully agreed.

I explained energy cleansings and performed a series of them on Emma's aura. She said she felt a little lighter and more grounded afterward, and she liked the smell of the lavender floral water I used. Next, I explained that she needed to extract some obstructing energies from her body. I sat her on a large cushion in front of the altar, and guided her in using my black extraction stone to remove them. After a few minutes,

Emma reported that she didn't know what came out, but it felt very heavy in her arm and then in the stone by the time she finished. I directed her to release these dense energies into the ground through my altar space.

Following the extraction, I gave Emma an overview of entities and how to identify them. As I guided her through the removal process, she located and expelled three irksome creatures. The first one, connected with her feeling of not being good enough, resisted the process but was eventually removed when we promised not to harm it. The second entity had been living in her knee, causing chronic pain ever since she had undergone knee surgery five years previously. It happily left with the guide.

Emma described the final one as having its claws in her shoulders, and it proved to be an angry being. When we addressed it, the entity moved around in Emma's body, trying to evade the process. Once detected, however, there was no escape, and the guides were able to remove the being and take it away. Emma said she felt calmer and more spacious once the entities were gone. I directed her to ask Source to fill the spaces vacated by the entities with whatever energies she wanted to replace them. She reported that she had the sensation of being filled with light, beauty and peace.

Next, I gave Emma a brief description of the shamanic journey, for which she decided to lie down. I darkened the room and led her down the steps into the unconscious and through the gateway. I then directed her to call in a higher guide, and she noted that a large light being appeared instantly. We determined that the being was of the light and appropriate for the journey, and I suggested Emma ask to see the inception of her suicidal feelings.

Shortly, Emma reported that she was seeing a scene of a family of four in what appeared to be a living room. We asked the guide if this was one of Emma's past lives. "No," he replied, so I encouraged her to ask who the people were. He informed her that the woman was her grandfather's oldest sister and that her name was Alice. The luminous being explained that Alice had recently been diagnosed with cancer, which had already metastasized throughout her body. Alice had not been feeling well for quite some time but had not gone to the doctor until the pain was unbearable.

The guide told Emma that Alice had just informed her husband and her two young sons about her cancer and prognosis. Emma told me she could see that Alice was despondent and extremely upset by the diagnosis and was very frightened to be facing a painful death. Alice's doctor had told her there were no treatment options available; there was nothing anyone could do for her. Emma said she could relate to Alice's feelings of utter despair and hopelessness. The husband and young sons were deep in fear and grief as well, knowing that Alice would soon succumb to this illness. They were unable to offer her any emotional support, and therefore Alice was all alone in her misery.

The light being then showed Emma how this story unfolded. The following morning, Alice arose before dawn while everyone was fast asleep. Emma watched as Alice— still in her nightgown but wrapped in an overcoat—made her way to the railway station several blocks from their home. Emma told me she already knew what was coming as the scene continued before her. Alice resolutely walked past the end of the station and hid behind an outbuilding. As the high-speed train approached, it was clear that it would not stop at the station. Mere seconds before the train reached her location, Alice stepped out from behind the building and into the locomotive's path. Emma said the scene went dark at that point, sparing her the sight of the grisly death. We were both feeling the horror of this event and stopped for a few minutes to let it settle.

The death was reported in the newspaper the next day as a suicide, describing that Alice had intentionally stepped in front of the early morning train. However, within two days, the same newspaper called it a "tragic accident" with no mention of suicide. The husband, distraught and devastated, could not endure the pain and stigma of suicide, living in a small town where everyone knew what had happened. The guide revealed that the suicide, and much of the grieving process, had been swept under the rug. The family never talked about this tragic event, and no one in town did, either. No one mentioned Alice's name again, and she disappeared from the family's reality.

Emma's grandfather, George, and the extended family were deeply traumatized by the event and also chose to bury it. George adored his big sister and had always felt a special connection with her, but he never again spoke of Alice or her death. The spirit guide then revealed the archived shock George had carried in his body until he died. Emma said she saw this as an "energy deposit" that contained the suppressed trauma of the suicide.

The guide showed Emma that her mother had inherited this same trauma energy bundle, and she could see where it had resided in her mother's body until her death. The luminous being then disclosed that Emma had received the packet in the same way and showed her where it was embedded in her body. Emma now understood that this archive held the imprint or record of the entire traumatic event, "like a sequestered file passed down the family lineage" until someone consciously addressed it.

Emma then remarked that "the file had become active" in her, which she thought was because of her sensitivity. "Or maybe the time was right for it to emerge for healing," she added. Emma described seeing how the imprint of the trauma unfolded in her life as part of her emotional nature. She gasped as she realized that her lifelong suicidal impulses were not hers but instead belonged to Alice. I urged her to confirm this with her guide, who said it was indeed true.

Next, I directed Emma to ask if she could return this suicidal energy to Alice, and the spirit helper replied, "Yes, you may." I suggested that Emma request her guide to bring Alice into the journey, which she then did. The light being immediately brought Alice in, and Emma reported that she could see that Alice was "in some kind of bubble or envelope." My impression was that this bubble was a *bardo* or mind realm and that Alice had been stuck in it because she committed suicide.

When Emma asked her guide about this, he confirmed that Alice had been in this bubble since her death. She then asked the spirit helper to transfer the suicidal energy bundle back to Alice, which he completed instantly. Emma remarked that as soon as Alice received this energy, she noticeably changed. I asked Emma what she was seeing, and she replied, "Alice looks more animated and even relieved!" We both thought this was an interesting response to what we considered to be toxic and traumatic energy.

I then recommended that Emma ask if we could request celestial assistance to help Alice get out of her bardo and on with her evolutionary path. The guide replied that we could petition for this assistance. I sensed that Archangel Michael would be an optimal choice and suggested this to Emma, who agreed wholeheartedly. She voiced her request aloud to Archangel Michael, and he immediately appeared. He completely cleared the bubble from around Alice and escorted her through an ethereal portal into a very bright light. As this was happening, both Emma and I felt electric tingles throughout our bodies, which Emma accurately described as "feeling glory." The glowing doorway neatly closed behind them, and they were gone.

We were both greatly affected by this, and Emma enthusiastically thanked Archangel Michael for his service. I recommended that she ask her spirit guide to fill the space where the energy packet had been with the energies of her choice, and she responded that he had filled her body and energy field with love.

I asked Emma how she felt after this intense experience, to which she replied, "I feel energized and optimistic about my life." She knew that Alice's suicidal feelings were gone and was relieved to understand that they had never even been her feelings at all. I told her I was grateful and deeply impressed by this powerful healing.

Next, I suggested Emma ask if there was anything else for us to address, and her guide advised us that we had done enough for the day. Emma asked to return to the gateway, which instantly occurred. She then thanked the luminous being for healing Alice and herself and said she was ready to end the journey. I brought her back through the gateway, up the steps and into our everyday reality.

I opened the curtains as Emma sat up and oriented herself. She always looked good, yet now there was a new lightness and sparkle about her. She was fascinated by what she had seen and experienced, adding that, as strange as it seemed, it all made perfect sense to her. She said she was elated that she had given the suicidal energy back to Alice and, even more, helped Alice move on to her next stage of life. "It was like witnessing magic," she said. "I never imagined it would be anything like what I experienced." I told her I felt inspired by the healing and that it had been a novel experience for me, too. We chatted about her journey for a while, and then I filled her aura with luminous energy and prayers. After ensuring that she was grounded and present, we thanked our guides and closed the sacred space for the day.

I checked in with Emma several months later, and she told me her suicidal feelings were indeed gone. She had not thought about suicide since the day of her shamanic journey and thanked me again for facilitating her healing experience. She shared that she now frequently awoke feeling filled with gratitude and vitality, still in awe that those lifelong feelings had never been hers.

* * *

The changes that occur as a result of this healing work on one's ancestors are profound and lasting for the living, and one can only assume that they also heal the departed. It helps to remember that our ancestors still exist and we are all eternally connected. As the ancient art of ancestral healing and honoring is reawakening in our Western culture, more people are becoming aware of this body of wisdom and dedicating time and energy to integrating it into their lives. These actions will affect the collective in many positive ways, in addition to healing individual lives.

A corollary to the work of ancestral healing that is also experiencing a much-needed revival is the art of helping people to die well. The aging and the passing of the Baby Boomers expose an enormous unmet need in our society. The inability to die well can be a source of problems for the living and a burden for the departing person. Our medical system's penchant for not informing an individual that they are about to die, or are in the process of dying, is an enormous disservice to the dying and their families. Fortunately, this misguided practice is slowly changing as doctors become more enlightened. Sometimes, people who do not die well can end up being earthbound spirits—often referred to as ghosts—who then have trouble moving on.

The following case study deals with ancestors whose trauma had blocked their ability to progress to other realms. These ancestors appeared to be farther back in the past and carried embedded trauma that they had not resolved, which kept them stuck in suspended animation. This condition is reminiscent of the lost fragments encountered in soul retrievals. A living person sometimes has a feeling, a dream or visitation from an ancestor or guide indicating that the ancestor requires assistance. Linda described receiving this kind of intuitive message that came unexpectedly one day.

* * *

Linda had been referred by a friend and contacted me to ask if I could help her do some healing work with her ancestors. She stated that she had not done this type of work previously but had concerns about several ancestors needing some kind of help. I asked if she had more information and knew who these ancestors were, to which she replied that she did not have any names and didn't know much about her genealogy. She had done some online research that described how a person could heal their ancestors but decided that she needed in-person guidance. Because of her feelings, she believed that her ancestors needed healing and that she was the one to accomplish it. I told her we very likely could help her ancestors through the shamanic journey work.

I oriented Linda to my healing room. She was a petite older woman with long, salt-and-pepper hair and a solemn expression. I introduced her to my altar, explaining that it would assist us in the work we would do. She mentioned that she could feel pleasant energy emanating from it. Together, we opened sacred space and called in our spiritual support, and I then outlined the process we would follow. She was knowledgeable about guided meditation and excited to participate in a journey. I began with the series of aura energy cleansings, which she said she could distinctly feel, even though there was not much for me to remove.

I sensed Linda was clear of obstructing entities so we moved directly into the shamanic journey. I recommend that she lie down, put on a blindfold and begin to relax. Then I led her down the steps, through the gateway and directed her to call in a higher guide. She announced that an angelic-looking being immediately appeared, and we verified that the guide was of the light.

I suggested she also call for a benevolent and healthy ancestor to come in. She said that as she did this, a rather strange-looking being appeared. He indicated that he was not of the light, so we quickly sent him away. Linda again called for a benevolent ancestor, and this time a woman appeared. Her name was Norma, and she assured us that she was Linda's ancestor and was of the light. We decided to work with both Norma and the higher guide to facilitate the healing journey.

Next, I directed Linda to ask Norma if there was any ancestral healing that we could carry out. Linda did so but reported that Norma did not respond to this question. I suggested we rephrase it, asking if there was ancestral healing that we were permitted to do for recent ancestors, going back no more than 500 years. In answer to that question, Norma immediately brought in four of Linda's ancestors.

We asked Norma on whom we should start, and she brought the first person forward. Norma explained the situation to Linda in great detail. The woman, named Bryn, had died a great many years ago, but recently enough for our work. A man with a spear had killed Bryn and thrown her corpse into a lake to hide the deed. Norma explained that Bryn "was stuck in limbo" because of her murder and could not move on. I asked if this limbo could be the same thing as a bardo, and Norma replied that they were the same. Linda could see that Bryn had two strong attachments, or energy fields, that were keeping her stuck.

Firstly, Bryn wanted justice for her murder and secondly, she was intensely worried about her four young children. Linda described Bryn as being "encapsulated" in these ensnaring energies and unable to free herself from them. I suggested Linda call upon her guide to address the issue of the children first. The angel showed Bryn some scenes of her children, both immediately after their mother's death and then again at several points much later in their lives. Linda said the children had all survived and had done well as they grew older. The experience of seeing her children thriving appeared to give Bryn a great deal of peace, and Linda could see some of the encapsulation around Bryn begin to dissipate.

I then urged Linda to ask to see all the circumstances around the murder. Bryn had been out gathering herbs at night in the countryside. A "Viking-like man" suddenly appeared on the scene and killed her with his spear. This act was seemingly random, done purely for the lust of killing, and Linda and I both found this senseless murder to be gruesome and disturbing. We asked the spirit guide to continue to reveal what happened in this story.

Linda proceeded, saying that eventually, this man had deep guilt and remorse for killing an innocent woman. This revelation by the higher guide of the murderer's feelings helped ease Bryn's bitterness at being killed, and her encapsulation diminished slightly more. As time progressed, the man immersed himself in genuine penance for the killing by trying to make other people's lives better. Linda said she could see this helped Bryn feel that her death had not been meaningless, and the encasement further dissipated.

Next, I suggested that Linda ask her guide to tell Bryn that she was member of Bryn's lineage and allow Bryn to perceive her. The angel agreed and explained to Bryn that Linda was one of her distant descendants. Linda was quite startled when Bryn came very close and intently looked at her. She allowed Bryn to examine her and experience her energy. Linda then spontaneously told Bryn how grateful she was that Bryn was her ancestor and sincerely thanked her, all of which markedly brightened Bryn's spirit.

I encouraged Linda to speak prayers of forgiveness, compassion, love and light for Bryn's sacrifice. We both felt these prayers enter deeply into Bryn, and Linda observed that the encapsulation had dissolved completely with the prayers. At last, Bryn was no longer a prisoner of her attachments. Linda was surprised as Bryn again came close and gave her a gift—a gold box lined with red velvet. She thanked Bryn and put this box inside herself for safekeeping. I then suggested Linda ask her guide to please escort Bryn out of limbo and into the light. Linda watched as a higher-dimensional portal opened and several glowing beings appeared. These shining ones gently led Bryn through the gateway, where they all disappeared as it closed behind them.

Norma then brought in the second ancestor, whom Linda described as a "raggedy woman locked in a gloomy dungeon" who was crawling about on a dirty stone floor. Linda felt that this poor soul was slowly starving to death and said she knew the woman had died in that dungeon. She then realized that this ancestor, too, was trapped in a mental realm of her misery. Her name was Gwendolyn, and we asked Norma to show us more details of her plight. With shock and disgust, Linda said there was an enormous vile creature with huge hands gripping Gwendolyn. This being would not release the woman and was torturing her mercilessly.

Linda asked the higher guide if we could help Gwendolyn, and she replied that we could. I suggested that Linda request the angel to remove the sinister energies that were surrounding Gwendolyn. The spirit guide immediately cleared the oppressive atmosphere from the dungeon, but the unsavory being remained. I recognized that it was an entity and that we needed Archangel Michael to remove its tenacious grip, so I recommended Linda call upon him aloud. Archangel Michael appeared and "took most of the creature away, except for the hands." Linda was dismayed to see the two huge hands still clinging to her ancestor and terrorizing her.

I then directed Linda to call upon the Cosmic Christ for assistance. She requested aloud that the Cosmic Christ please come in and entirely remove the hands of the entity. With that, a radiant orb of light appeared and took the hands away, completely freeing Gwendolyn. At that same moment, both Linda and I felt our hearts fill with vibrant love and light, and we both thanked Archangel Michael and the Cosmic Christ for assisting us.

Once Gwendolyn was freed from the thought-form, we sent her compassion, forgiveness, self-acceptance and healing prayers. Linda then asked her guide to transport Gwendolyn out of the miserable dungeon and into the light, allowing her to move on. At that moment, several towering angelic beings appeared, picked Gwendolyn up and carried her through a luminous portal, which closed behind them and vanished. We paused for a few moments to assimilate this intense episode.

Noor was the third ancestor that Norma brought in, explaining to Linda that she had been a young mother whose baby died shortly after birth. Noor was bereft and inconsolable over the loss, and her grief had immobilized her. I suggested we ask the guide to show Noor an expanded view of her entire life. Linda described this as "looking at a diorama of Noor's lifetime." In this enlarged scene, Noor was able to witness that this infant's soul had returned to her; the next child Noor conceived and birthed was this very same being. Linda reported that, as Noor took in the entire cycle of life and death and life, she appeared to be immensely relieved and more accepting of the situation.

However, Noor still could not let go of the grief she had been holding so tightly. Linda said she could see this grief as "a complex of energy, like a web" that kept Noor stuck. I suggested Linda call upon Ascended Master Saint Germain to help her, which she did. He immediately appeared, and I directed her to request that he please lift the grief and suffering from Noor and transmute it into light. A scintillating violet flame entered both of our perceptions as he accomplished this transmutation. Linda reported that Noor's heart had been cleared and then filled with light and peace. We both thanked Saint Germain for this healing, and he departed.

Noor was now smiling, free from the web and ready to move on, so I asked Linda to call upon Noor's guides to assist her. As she did, several lofty spirit beings came in and took Noor away with them. Sensations of deep peace and harmony filled both of us at the resolution of Noor's grief and her ascension into the light.

Norma then presented the final ancestor for the healing session. Linda described seeing a very young boy whose dog had recently died. With the trauma of the dog's death, a piece of the boy, whose name was Toshi, had split off. Linda realized that it was this fragment of the young Toshi that was sitting on a stone grieving his dead dog. The rest of Toshi had gone on to live out his earthly life; he had grown up, married, had a family, and eventually became Linda's distant ancestor.

I suggested we do a soul retrieval for Toshi, and Linda asked her guide for assistance. First, the angel brought the dog back to life, which restored joy and animation to the grieving soul fragment. Next, she reinstated the small-boy piece of Toshi back into the grown man. Linda said she could see the healing energy of this reunion rippling through his entire being, extending throughout his lifetime, and restoring his wholeness. She exclaimed that this process both looked and felt miraculous. Norma then advised us that Toshi's healing was complete and took him back to wherever he belonged. When she reappeared, Norma stated that we had completed our session. We thanked her for all her help in healing Linda's ancestors, at which point she smiled, nodded and departed.

I then asked Linda to have her higher guide take her back to the gateway, and she replied that she was instantly there. She thanked the angel for her masterly assistance, to which her guide responded that she would always be there whenever Linda called. When they finished speaking, I asked Linda if she was ready to return and brought her back into our consensual reality.

Linda expressed her awe and profound gratitude for the opportunity to do such important work. She said her experiences in the session made her heart lighter and that, somehow, she felt healed for having experienced it. I noted that she did seem lighter, and her serious expression had softened considerably. I told her I was pleased with the extensive healing we had done and encouraged her to continue doing this kind of work with the help of both Norma and her angelic guide. She thanked me for the encouragement and said she was looking forward to embarking on another ancestral journey. We then ended the session, thanking the guides and closing our sacred space.

* * *

Most often, I encounter a mixture of the categories of ancestors mentioned above. Using the shamanic journey process, the practitioner can seamlessly transition from one healing episode, issue or problem to the next. The higher guides are adept at ancestral healing, and the healthy and luminous ancestors can become our spiritual allies, as Norma had been in the case study above. It is essential to work with beings who are of the light to obtain superior results. Our healthy ancestors can also be vital resources for personal healing and more. In his book *Ancestral Medicine,* Daniel Foor states that "…on a cultural and collective level, the ancestors are powerful allies in transforming historical trauma relating to race, gender, religion, war and other types of collective pain."[6]

Ancestral healing is powerful work, and as we do more of it as a culture, we will see our collective consciousness heal and shift. Many of us were born into fragmented and dysfunctional families carrying unresolved trauma from multiple past generations. Ancestor healing work can directly and successfully address this trauma. However, we must begin with understanding the importance of focusing on one's healthy ancestors and requesting their assistance with this healing. As Dr. Foor describes, "We all have loving and supportive ancestors and can draw upon these relationships for greater clarity about life purpose, increased health and vitality, and tangible support in daily life."[7] Building relationships with our ancestors can be a two-way street since the living can help the ancestors and the ancestors can assist the living, healing the entire lineage and, as an extension, humanity.

At times, we might encounter ancestors who are not whole and well, and therefore cannot consider them as allies. Troubled ancestors may draw energy from the living and can be a source of "bad luck" or other challenges for their descendants. Such a situation might be convoluted and difficult to unravel, and the healing that is needed may be more than the client wishes to undertake. In some cases, what is inherited can be the result of curses and dark energies, as we saw in Marisol's case study.

Chapter 8

Entities and Entity Removal

ONE FACTOR THAT MAKES WORKING with entities challenging is that we, culturally, do not believe in such things. Entities are generally classified as old wives' tales or witchcraft, ridiculed and summarily dismissed as a figment of someone's imagination or mental disorder. I have a shamanic perspective on these beings based on many years of direct experience with my clients. In countless cases, longstanding physical, emotional, mental and spiritual problems have immediately resolved once the entity was identified and evicted. The probability that these conditions cleared because of some imaginative or placebo effect is negligible since the procedure is nearly one hundred percent effective.

What do I mean by the nebulous term *entities?* As I mentioned previously, these can be embedded thought-forms, beliefs, emotional and behavioral conditioning, or other energy constructs and can also be disembodied or nonphysical beings of various types. Indigenous peoples might call them evil spirits. The pertinent identifier for entities is that they are alive, conscious and can communicate with us; thus, they are sentient creatures of some kind. Among my clients, I have found entities to be very common, and every person, to some extent, likely has had these energetic beings living in them at one time or another.

As conscious nonphysical beings, entities can affect and influence the human they inhabit without actually controlling them. The entity may also identify itself as an aspect of the person it is inhabiting, which may or may not be true. The currently popular Internal Family Systems approach to psychotherapy describes how many people have multiple "parts" that make up the whole of a person's psyche. Some people may have very active internal "parts" that have dissociated and can present as an entity. An entity can also be blended with a "part" of a person, making it challenging to differentiate who and what is there. I have also encountered a few deceased human spirits dwelling within clients, which may at first appear to be an entity. Once a being has been identified, it can be asked if it is a "part" of the person or if it is a deceased human. It is best not to ask it if it is an entity, since many entities do not know what they are, and they can, and do, lie. Generally, the response is true and the practitioner can proceed accordingly. If the answer received is not clear, or seems untrue, a guide can be invoked to provide clarity. If it is a "part" of the person, the higher guide can confirm this, and help to reintegrate the "part" back into the person as a whole, or give specific advice about it to the client. If it is a deceased human, the spirit guide can open a portal and escort the being on to their next phase of life. Depending on the client, this can be done as part of the entity removal process, or may need to be done within the guided shamanic journey.

There is another possibility which I consider to be possession. I define *possession* as a malevolent force or being that has taken control over a living human in an unsolicited and unwelcome manner. This does not include the practice of channeling, or possession for the purpose of oracular divination or healing that is practiced in some spiritual traditions. These external spiritual invaders can range from merely troublesome to extremely demonic and come in many forms, yet a common feature is their refusal to depart. Deceased human spirits, or ghosts, on the other hand, can influence a person but usually do not possess them, taking over the life and free will of the client. In my experience, true possession is rare. Calling in a possession specialist guide or higher levels of spiritual helpers to remedy this condition is the best way to proceed.

Entities can block, suppress or alter the healthy energy flow in the human body, either purposefully or unintentionally. They become an issue when they begin to create problems, such as chronic pain, mental or emotional distress, or physical dis-ease. Many clients who have come to me with chronic pain have had entities connected to that pain. The pain either resolves immediately (if it was entirely due to the entity) or greatly diminishes (if there was also an underlying physical condition) when the entity is expelled. I have observed that it is common for people who have undergone surgery of any kind or have had long stays in a hospital to be carrying entities.

How do you know if you have an entity? There appear to be a wide variety of symptoms indicating an entity might be present, and these run the gamut between mild and extreme. Some examples are obsessive thoughts, addictions, depression, suicidal thoughts, panic attacks, nightmares, feeling spacey, lack of concentration, hearing voices, extreme fatigue, long-term anger or sudden and drastic behavior change. There can be many other causes of these same symptoms, so it is essential to delve specifically into each case. It is a quick and easy matter to conduct the entity removal process and, if no entity is discovered, that is not the cause of the problem. There is no downside to doing this simple, noninvasive process.

Fortunately, we do not need to know precisely what entities are, or where they come from, to work with them. Most people can communicate directly with the entity in some way when guided to do so. A few clients have recognized their entity and acknowledged having had a relationship with it for years, some since childhood. When I question them about this, they admit that they never stopped to think about what the voice they were hearing might be. People often believe this voice is simply speaking their thoughts to them, which is especially true if the creature has been present for many years, or is actually a "part" of them.

Over the decades, I have come to view certain entities as relatively benign beings who want to experience embodied life. Since they lack a physical incarnation of their own, they must await opportunities to enter and become incorporated into a human body. Usually, once they have become embodied, they want to stay. However, the entity is trespassing and does not have a right to continue to occupy that physical body. It can only remain with the person's permission; without that permission, it must leave when told to do so. Some entities, however, can be very resistant.

How do entities enter someone? I have observed a variety of methods: they may be invited in by the person (usually in early childhood); they may enter when a person is unconscious due to surgery, an accident or coma; they can also gain access when the person has passed out or lost consciousness for some other reason. Anyone who practices shamanic journeying or out-of-body travel, and doesn't adequately protect their body while they are out, can allow an entity to come in during their absence. I believe that entities and deceased human spirits can even be inherited. A recent client had a deceased ancestor who did not know he was dead. He had been passed down for what he termed "many generations" until we contacted him. Once we informed him that he was no longer alive on the earth plane, he was delighted to be escorted through the portal into the spirit realm. The main problem is that entities are able to stay because their presence remains unknown to the person who has them—or, even if the individual does suspect it, they may not know how to remove the creatures.

Most entities can be easily expelled once they are detected, so the key is to identify them as invaders in the first place. I have read that some energy workers kill entities, which I think is unethical. How can anyone possibly know what function entities serve in the grand scheme of things? They are alive and conscious, are part of All That Is, and therefore have a purpose. Even malevolent entities have a purpose and reason for being and, as I have mentioned, appear to be more common now than in previous years. These hostile beings can be extremely damaging, and the person must remove them to heal fully. The following unusual case study includes interactions with several malicious entities.

* * *

Beth was a young woman who was in the midst of a real crisis. Her aunt, who was a student of shamanism, had called me as soon as Beth was admitted to the hospital to discuss the symptoms Beth was having. She was convinced that Beth did not have a psychiatric condition but was filled with entities, and she wanted my opinion. We talked for quite some time and I told her that, based on what she was telling me, I agreed that entities could be responsible for her behavior. I offered to see Beth once she was released if the family agreed.

A few days later, Beth's mother, who was her advocate, called to make an appointment upon Beth's release from the hospital. I interviewed her mother extensively to determine the underlying problem, and she narrated a story that began several months previously with Beth hearing voices. Beth had finally told her concerned mother that there were multiple voices and that they were abusive, loud, and hostile. Beth could not shut them up. These voices pestered her day and night, saying bizarre things to her and influencing her to commit strange and dangerous acts. Beth thought that these voices were an aspect of herself because they told her they were, and she was unable to separate herself from them.

Over time, Beth began agreeing with the voices and doing the things they suggested, but she did not tell anyone what was happening. Gradually, the voices became more belligerent and hostile, completely blocking out her everyday life. This affliction ultimately led to Beth putting a lighted cigarette out on her forehead when the voices insisted on it. This act resulted in a nasty wound and exposed the problem to Beth's anxious mother, who immediately took her to the emergency room.

Beth was treated in the ER and then questioned at length about how she had managed to burn herself on her forehead. Based on the answers she gave them, the doctors determined that Beth was both bipolar and schizophrenic. They entered these diagnoses in her medical record and promptly admitted her to the psych ward for six weeks. The doctors also administered three powerful psychoactive drugs to control her conditions and ordered psychiatric follow-up assessments for her each week.

As part of my inquiry into Beth's history, her mother told me Beth was a gifted healer in a talented family but had been traumatized in childhood and had many unresolved problems. She disclosed that Beth had been raped at age four and had had a series of other sexual assaults over the years. Beth had been in therapy for many years to heal from this abuse and seemed to be doing well. Her mother reiterated that she had not known about all the voices until the cigarette episode happened, which deeply worried her. She had contacted me on the advice of her sister who felt confident I could resolve the issue, and she pointedly asked me if I thought I could help Beth once she was released. I told her that I was sure Beth was carrying entities that we could remove, and we set a date for the session.

After the six weeks had passed, Beth was released into her mother's care, with the provision of attending weekly psychiatric appointments to monitor her medications. The medications had done nothing to silence the voices, and they continued unabated. Beth, slender and petite with sandy brown hair and a somber expression, arrived with her mother for the session. I escorted them both into my healing room and asked Beth if she wanted her mother to stay. She replied that she did, to which her silver-haired mother agreed. I asked them both many more questions about Beth's experiences. Since Beth was very subdued because of the intense medications, her well-informed and articulate mother provided much of the information I needed.

I oriented Beth to my altar, where she would be sitting. She loved the balance, stability and peace she said emanated from it. I invited them both to join me in opening sacred space and calling in our spiritual support. They were unfamiliar with energy work, so I gave them an overview of how we would proceed. Beth agreed to participate as much as possible since I had explained that it was a critical part of the process. Beth's mother then took a seat on a cushion to the north of the altar.

With Beth standing next to my altar, I began with the series of energy cleansings on her aura, observing that she was keenly sensitive to energetic work. Despite her medication-dampened emotions, she was acutely feeling each step as I removed many layers of thick, sticky energy. I then pulled more of this tarry energy out of the burn scar on her forehead and from her heart center, using a crystal from my altar, and discharged this energy into my altar ground.

Next, I had Beth sit directly in front of the altar and pick up my black tourmaline. I guided her to remove the dense energy from inside her body by using the extraction process. Beth reported that she felt a large amount of heavy, putrid energy coming out of her body and into the stone. I told her to release that energy into the ground by blowing forcefully on the stone toward the floor. I then taught her how to cleanse the tool with rue water. When she finished the extraction process, she said she already felt much better.

We then moved on to address the sinister entities I knew were there. I explained the concept of entities to Beth and outlined what we would be doing to remove them. She quickly grasped what I was describing and had no problem contacting them, as these were the disturbing voices she was hearing. Due to her extraordinary perceptive abilities, she could hear and interact with the entities much more directly than most people. Unfortunately, this heightened sensitivity also made her more susceptible to their negative influences. I explained this to her so she wouldn't blame herself for being too sensitive and would focus on the task at hand.

The first entity Beth encountered was very malicious and stubborn and was clearly one of the abusive voices in her mind. It refused to comply, telling her to "just give it up" because it was not leaving. I explained to Beth that the entity, regardless of what it said, had no right to occupy her body and asked her if she wanted to be free of it. She replied that she was determined to remove it and asked me to help her. It took both my guidance and considerable help from the guides to expel this tenacious and cruel being. Once the unwelcome presence was gone, she announced that it was considerably quieter in her head, and she felt there was now more room for herself.

Beth quickly located a second entity and said it had "the energy of a young girl." She thought this was part of her inner child and questioned whether we should remove it. I explained to her that this is where the process can be very subjective. I distinctly felt it as an entity and guided her to ask it specific questions. Listening to the answers it gave, we both agreed that it was not her inner child or a part of her. I directed her to tell the young girl energy that it was not part of her. Upon hearing that, the entity said, "Oh, okay," and was very willing to leave with the guides. This being was apparently just as confused as Beth about its identity and immediately vacated her body.

Beth sensed that a third entity was present, but it was elusive and difficult to pin down. She recognized it as the voice that always told her to doubt herself. It also stated that it was unwilling to leave, and I reminded Beth that this was not an option because it was not up to the entity to decide. We promised it that we would not harm it and would help it go onward, and the being finally released its stubborn grip. Beth called in the guides, who succeeded in taking it away.

After expelling these three entities, Beth felt a great deal better and commented that the headaches she usually had were completely gone. She pointed to her lower left occipital region and said, "Yes, I can feel that this area is now clear." Beth did not detect any other entities, so we decided to move on, but I told her I felt sure that more would appear over time.

I then explained the purpose and process of the guided shamanic journey. Beth chose to lie down on a pad on the floor beside my altar and began to relax as I darkened the room. I led her down the steps into the unconscious and directed her to call in her master-healer guide. The spirit being who instantly appeared confirmed her service to the light. I suggested that Beth ask if she had cording to anyone that we could remove now. Her guide replied that there was only one person who would be relevant for this session, and she immediately brought the person, in their etheric body, to face Beth.

I walked Beth through the cord removal process. Being very skilled at perceiving nonphysical energies, she easily located and dismantled the cords both from herself and the other person. Once she removed them, I directed her to transmute them into light. The person was then escorted away, and the guide told Beth that although she had cording with many more people, this was the only one we could work with today.

Next, I recommended Beth ask if there were any fragments of herself that we could retrieve. The luminous guide stated that there was one we could address at present. I advised Beth to ask to go to that fragment, and she said she was now looking at a very young aspect of herself. When we asked the soul piece if it wanted to return, it indicated that it was not sure. I explained to Beth that this piece of herself had been in suspended animation since the trauma that had cleaved it off, so it did not know who Beth was now. I told her she needed to tell the fragment what had happened in her life since it split and bring it up to the present moment. Beth assured the small fragment that she was now a grown woman and her life was very different than it had been. The young piece listened closely to her words but was still unsure what to do.

I proposed that Beth ask the fragment if it was willing to come into my body first and then go into hers. The soul piece agreed to this option and, without hesitation, came into my body. I felt it as light energy, welcomed it by sending it love, and gave it time to adjust to being in a body. Then I asked if it was ready to go back into Beth's body, which it said it now was. I blew the soul fragment back into Beth's heart chakra and told her to welcome it. Beth said she could feel it as part of her and was delighted to have it back. She noted that it felt very different than the entity that had seemed to be part of her. I explained the importance of caring for this piece of herself and making sure her young fragment felt welcome and loved. Beth understood and agreed to do this.

The guide then advised Beth that we were finished and would need to do the rest of the work in another session. I told Beth to request to be returned to the gateway and said she was there. I urged her to ask her master healer if she would be available to Beth for healing journeys that Beth could do on her own. The spirit helper assured her she would always be present for continuing this work and more. Beth was delighted to hear this and said she would call on her guide often. I encouraged Beth to work directly with this luminous being at every opportunity and reminded her to thank the guide for all she had facilitated. Then, when Beth was ready, I brought her up from the gateway to the unconscious and into my healing space.

I asked Beth how she felt, and she replied that she was feeling much happier and lighter than when she arrived and was more hopeful than she had been in many months. She was smiling and more animated than she had been, and her somber expression had softened. I reminded her that there were more entities than the ones we had expelled and that they would surface from time to time in everyday life. I asked her and her mother if they would be able to follow the entity removal on their own, to which they both replied, "Yes."

I then told Beth I suspected she had a tear or hole in her aura that had allowed these exceptionally harmful entities to enter her body. Her response shocked me. "Oh, yes," she said, "I have a large tear in my aura right here," and she pointed to an arc of space above her head that extended down her neck and into her back. I do not usually see auras, but Beth could vividly see hers, as well as the hole in it. When I questioned her, she said she had been aware of the tear but thought nothing of it. I asked how she managed to get this extensive gash, and she responded that, not long before, she had "smoked PCP and DMT at a gathering with some friends." She stated that the damage had occurred during that episode.

When I recovered from my shock at this disclosure, Beth and I discussed at length why smoking these substances was extremely unwise, especially at a party. I explained that there are much better ways to work with altered states and plant medicine. She agreed that it had not been a good idea and promised she wouldn't do it again. I handed her a crystal tool from my altar and directed her to use it to sew up the split in her aura. She took the crystal and deftly stitched her torn aura back together. I then asked her to call on Archangel Michael and request that he come in and heal the gash. As Beth did so, she reported that she saw him appear and repair the damage, leaving her aura shimmering.

Beth was noticeably feeling better, and her eyes were shining as we talked about her journey experiences. I gave her specific instructions on how she could protect herself in the future. When we finished, I concluded the session by filling her energy field with high-vibration energies, using rose water, feathers and prayers. I reminded her and her mother that there was still a lot of healing work to finish and that they needed to return in a few weeks for another session. As a homework assignment, I recommended that Beth set up a sacred altar at home and use it as a focal point for working with her master-healer guide, which she agreed to do. I again asked them if they thought they could do the entity and cord removal processes, and both expressed confidence that they could. We then thanked all our spiritual support and closed sacred space for the day. They thanked me again for helping them, and I could see expressions of relief on both of their faces.

* * *

Entity Removal Process

Overview:

The energy practitioner will have completed an in-depth interview with the client before the healing session. When discussing the process, the practitioner should be alert to the language the individual uses to describe themselves and the issues they want to address. Be aware of any symptoms that might be caused by an entity, keeping in mind that many other conditions can present in similar ways. Further investigation is always warranted, so I frequently begin by having my client directly address a particular symptom and see if it responds. If you uncover extreme responses, ask your client if they have a psychological diagnosis of any kind.

Potential symptoms of entities:

1. Obsessive thoughts, particularly hopeless or fearful ones
2. Addictions of any kind or starting a new bad habit
3. Long-term anger, resentment, judgment or blaming
4. Hearing a voice or voices
5. Physical, mental or emotional problems not responding to other treatment
6. Problems with thinking, remembering or concentrating; feeling very spacey

7. Depression, suicidal thoughts, or panic attacks
8. Drastic behavior changes within a short timeframe
9. Unexplained loss of energy, extreme fatigue, or disconnection from life
10. 10. Nightmares; being chased in dreams; feeling attacked or persecuted

It is essential to understand that this process is not a dialogue or a negotiation. It is a decree that expels the entity. As mentioned, entities can be malevolent, deceitful and even persuasive if they do not want to leave. They can deceive or shape-shift to appear as something else; they can even release subtle energies into the room to manipulate the situation.

After your client has arrived, open your sacred space (including grounding) and call in spiritual support for the healing process. Perform a series of energy cleansings to remove all obstructing energies from the client's aura, followed by a stone extraction removing any internalized harmful energy. I recommend that the practitioner complete the steps for entity removal before guiding anyone into the shamanic journey. Some entities can be disruptive and cause unnecessary problems during any journey the client undertakes. If it is not possible to remove the entity beforehand, this method can be added to the journey format itself. When I sense that my client might have a problem with the word *entity*, I use another term, such as *thought-form* or *introject*.

When my client is ready to begin, I have them sit at my sacred altar, which provides spiritual support for the healing process. If you do not have an altar, it is best to be in a setting that feels clean, safe and sacred. I ensure that the person feels comfortable, present, grounded and in their body before I begin.

I then ask them to focus on any pain, feelings, perceptions or sensations in the body that they are aware of at the moment. I explain that these could be chronic aches and pains, feelings of tightness or constriction, negative self-talk, odd sensations in the body, fear, or any of the other symptoms listed above. Any energy that moves around inside someone's body is, I believe, always an entity—this is a common occurrence. For example, the person might say they feel knee pain and then suddenly say that it has moved and is now in their shoulder.

The identification aspect of the process can be a subtle and subjective experience for the client and practitioner alike, or it can be quite dramatic and intense. Anything that comes up during the session can be a clue about the dynamics of the situation and warrants addressing. It is vital that the client has a perception of the entity and can communicate with it during this process. Fortunately, most people can communicate in some manner with these beings.

Many entities might have been beneficial when they first entered the individual's body, especially if embodied during childhood. I believe that even innocuous entities will, over time, eventually cause dis-ease and problems for those they inhabit. As time passes, the entity increasingly identifies itself with the person, and the person does not realize that there is a foreign being inside them. Gradually, the entity attempts to direct the individual's life, give advice and make decisions for the host. It is this clash that frequently results in the symptoms that have emerged. At best, entities block the free and healthy flow of energies through the human physical and nonphysical bodies.

The practitioner needs to direct the entity removal procedure, at least initially. I have found that many people need me to repeat the entire process, word for word, with each entity encountered because they have difficulty focusing on and remembering the steps once they connect to the entity. The client must be willing to expel the being to heal the problem.

As with the shamanic journey, I always engage guides in the removal of entities. Every being appears to have a spirit guide who watches over them—no one is ever alone. Therefore, every entity has a guide who will facilitate its removal at the decree of the person it is inhabiting; however, higher guides cannot remove any entity without this direct request. The guide will then compassionately take the being away because they always know where to relocate it. Do not expel entities into the session space. In other words, do not leave entities in the environment where they can enter someone else. Always ask the guides to take them away. The guides will not remove a "part" of a person because they know it is a "part" and needs to be reintegrated. They will tell you this, if you ask.

Step-by-step process:

1. Once the client has identified a sensation, pain, symptom or movement, ask them to focus their attention on the place in their body where they feel it is located.

2. When they have focused their attention, tell them to say aloud to that place in their body, "What is your name?"

    The client then waits for a reply. Most commonly, they will receive a name or other response of some kind. This reply can be almost anything, so if there is one, follow it up. The names of entities appear to be arbitrary and usually not related to any human the client knows, even if it sounds like one they recognize.

    Ask the person to tell you every response they receive so you can monitor and facilitate the process. If there is no reply to that first question, simply continue with the process as described. Certain types of entities will typically hide and not answer questions, at least at first. Stay with the process, and the entity frequently will respond as you ask it more questions. If the client does not receive a name, you can address the energy as "entity" or "being."

3. Next, direct the client to say the name of the entity followed by: "You are an entity. You are not part of my body or energy field. Do you understand?"

    Usually, the entity will respond with a yes or no. Some entities know what they are, while others do not. I do not consider it worthwhile to delve into the entity's history, such as where it came from or how it entered the individual. If the entity has been with a person for a long time, possibly since childhood, it may no longer remember entering the person and might genuinely think it is the person. It is irrelevant whether the entity does or does not know what it is. Notifying it that it is an entity is what matters. If there is any doubt about it being an entity, now is the time to ask if it is a "part" of the client, or a deceased human spirit. In my experience, this is not common.

It's important to always ask the entity, "Do you understand?" This will help you get a sense of its attitude and give the client the direct experience of conversing with it. Whatever response is received, you then ask the person if they want to release this trespassing creature. If they do not, either proceed to locate other entities or end the process here. Otherwise, continue to the next step.

4. Ask the client to say aloud: "Entity, I am going to completely and permanently remove you from my body and energy field. Do you understand?"

Again, this usually results in a yes or no response from the entity, and by asking if it understands, you will gain additional insight into its "personality." If the entity is cruel, malicious, hostile, angry or resistant, it will usually make that clear to the person by the nature of its response. It may tell the person that they will not be able to get rid of it, that they will not be able to function without it, or that something unfortunate will happen to them if they do expel it. The entity might fear that it will die or be killed if it is removed. Many entities are willing to cooperate and go along with the process, so this is to be encouraged. If the entity is hesitant to comply, the following step frequently renders the entity more cooperative.

5. The client says aloud: "We are not going to harm you. We will ensure that you are taken where you need to go next, for your own evolution. Do you understand?"

Letting the entity know you will not harm it is a compassionate and helpful thing to do. Nearly all entities shift into a readiness to move on once they hear those words. If the person has anything they want to say to the entity before expelling it, this is the time to say it. By now, both the client and the entity should be ready to finish the process, and you can move to step 6. Note: If your client has not received any responses to the questions—particularly the last one—and neither you nor the client perceives an entity, there probably is none. You can either continue the process to detect other entities or move to another part of the session.

6. This step is the decree. Ask the client to say: "I call in the guides of this entity, and ask that you please come in and completely and permanently remove this entity from my body and energy field now!"

    This is said as a command, and includes the word "now." With this decree, the guides come in, remove the entity and take it wherever it needs to go. Frequently, the person can directly perceive this evacuation as it happens. They may feel instant relief from the originating symptoms or have a sense of more internal space, peace or stillness. Sometimes the client feels as if nothing has happened, and the practitioner must discern whether or not the entity is gone. In some cases, nothing has happened, and the entity is still embedded. If you did not previously ask if this is a "part" of the person, you might want to do that now. The guides will not remove a "part" because it belongs to client's greater Self.

    Occasionally, the guides either fail to remove or only partially remove the entity. Your client might report that "much" or "most" or "some" of the entity is gone. The guides who initially appear may not be able to remove the entity, in which case you need to call on another spirit helper who has more power. If an entity was not removed or only partially removed, I ask the client if they are familiar with Archangel Michael. Many people know of him, and some have worked with Archangel Michael for years. Others have no idea what an archangel is or don't believe in them. If they are unfamiliar with him, I explain that he is a very large and powerful angel with whom I work and that we will call him in to complete the removal.

7. If this step is needed, direct the client to say: "I call in Archangel Michael, and request that you please come in and completely and permanently remove this entity from my body and energy field now."

Most people can perceive the arrival of Archangel Michael at some level, and he nearly always removes the entity's remnants—or the entire entity, if necessary. On rare occasions, Archangel Michael is unable to remove the entire entity. I will then ask the client a series of questions to try to determine if they are holding on to it in any way. If they are, further explanation about entities and the problems they cause will generally help the person decide to release it. If Archangel Michael did not successfully remove it and the person is not holding on to the entity, I ask again if they want to expel it. If the answer is yes, we then proceed to an even more powerful helper.

8. Ask the client to say: "I call in Infinite Source Energy (or you can use 'the Cosmic Christ') and request that you please remove this entity completely and permanently now."

   This request has never failed unless the person is still holding on to the entity. Once it is gone, the client usually feels both a sense of relief and more spaciousness. They can then request that the higher guide fill any void created by the entity removal with light, love or other energies of their choosing.

9. Repeat the entire process as many times as necessary until no more entities are detected. It is common for clients to have more than one creature to expel. To conclude, ask your client how they are feeling now.

Chapter 9

Guided Shamanic Journey and Cord Removal

Guided shamanic journeys involve an imaginal tour of the unconscious using progressive relaxation and visualization, and shamanistic methods. This marriage of classic induction with shamanic journeying produces a successful technique for entering non-ordinary states to address and heal difficult conditions. The process is straightforward and can be finely tuned to specific questions or issues that we then place before the unlimited potentialities of the spiritual realms. The focus is to facilitate healing of physical, mental, emotional or spiritual dis-ease.

Progressive relaxation and visualization are well-known techniques used to help an individual enter a state of focused concentration, heightened suggestibility and reduced peripheral awareness. Guided visualization can also be used to facilitate deeper levels of perception. Whether this is an altered state or a form of active imagination is not the issue here. It is a deep exploration of the unconscious mind. We can use the journey process to obtain significant lasting results even if we do not thoroughly understand how it works. I have successfully used this technique with people who do not believe in a spiritual realm or altered states. I tell them that beliefs are irrelevant and rarely impede the journey experience. The simple process I use allows the client to enter into a very light trance where they can freely act under their own volition and communicate with me.

Each journey revolves around an individual's direct experience and interaction with spiritual guides, allowing us to resolve their specific conditions. Nearly everyone who approaches this process with an open mind and willingness to explore will have a self-evident experience traveling to other realities and receiving valuable healing assistance from their guides. In addition to any healing received, each person experiences a shift in their understanding and perspective, which may markedly expand their perception of reality and be therapeutic in itself.

Multiple healing issues may be addressed in a single session using classic shamanic and energy healing techniques. Many of these are highlighted in the case studies presented. Since energetic factors are present in virtually every form of illness, I encourage anyone who has not received relief from conventional medicine to utilize guided shamanic journeys to solicit information and assistance from the spirit realm. I have mentioned psychosomatic disorders, autoimmune illness, post-traumatic stress syndrome, obsessive-compulsive disorder, phobias and cancers as some of the conditions with powerful energetic components. Even diseases that have a physical basis nearly always have some form of unexamined emotional trauma embedded in them that can be directly addressed by higher beings.

We place the health conditions and other problems directly before the spirit guides and receive individualized responses appropriate to each person. The luminous beings have in-depth knowledge of the issues presented and how best to address them. The most important factor, in my mind, is that it is the client who journeys and has the direct experience of all that transpires. This is the opposite of the classic shamanic model where the shaman journeys, fixes the problem and returns to tell the person about it.

The practitioner focuses on the issues, comes up with questions for the guides and helps the client navigate the various realms of the unconscious. The higher guides generate the journey and facilitate all healing. The journeyer enjoys a direct perception of this entire process and gets to know their spirit helper. The practitioner never dictates specific experiences that the client will have and is just as surprised as anyone with the unfolding of the journey. I am frequently awed by the potency of healing that higher beings facilitate for my clients, and the brilliance of their solutions.

All higher guides engaged are intimately aware of the client's needs, history and life purpose. These light beings include a plethora of helping spirits and also a person's higher selves. There is both safety and unlimited potential in having Spirit do the energy healing work. The attending spirit beings determine what healing to perform and will guarantee that it is done properly and only at the request of the person seeking healing. They know everything about the client and all the potential outcomes that could unfold, which is entirely beyond our human capacity. I have also observed them giving incredibly insightful and loving counsel to their charges.

As I have mentioned, higher spiritual guides have explained that they are everyone, everywhere, at the same time, and thus know everything. They reside in Unity Consciousness, outside of time and space, unconstrained by third-dimensional physics. Frequently, I have witnessed them perform feats that appear to be utterly miraculous—and even beyond our ability to imagine.

Some clients can observe their guides and everything that happens during the shamanic journey, which is indeed fortunate. Others may have a knowing, sensations or feelings about what transpires, which is unique to them. Thus, any of a person's senses may be involved during the journey. However, direct perception of these events is not required for the healing to occur and be successful. Every journeyer personally communicates with their spirit helpers, and many can continue this direct communication even after the session has ended. Most people report having vivid and memorable experiences of everything that happened during the session and retain this memory upon returning to everyday awareness.

The case studies presented in this book contain examples of many conditions that can impact one's health. The same shamanic journey procedure may also be used to solve a variety of other problems and is not limited to health concerns.

* * *

As described in Chapter 8, Beth and her mother had consulted me regarding her tormenting voices. It was several weeks later that she and her mother met with me again. Beth appeared slightly more animated and present as I greeted them at the door. She quickly informed me that "the voices have returned," to which I replied that I was not surprised. She and her mother had removed three more entities between visits, but Beth was still troubled by voices. I congratulated them on expelling the creatures and assured them that we would get right to work on those that remained.

Beth and her mother joined me in standing at my altar as we opened sacred space and called in our spiritual support. Beth's mother took her seat on a cushion, and Beth remained standing for the cleansings. As I enacted the series of aura cleansings, I taught them both how to do each one. I strongly recommended that Beth perform this procedure daily, especially if she had been around many people. I then gave her several tools with which to continue the cleansings at home.

Next, I asked Beth to sit in front of my altar, and we turned our focus to the entities. As soon as we did this, Beth's mother, who was herself a healing practitioner, said she could see a shadowy figure on the back of Beth's neck and upper back. Neither Beth nor I could feel or sense it in any way. I directed Beth to address this shadow image and ask it its name. It refused to reply to the question, so I suggested that we continue by calling it "shadow energy," which Beth then did.

As we moved forward with the removal process, the entity suddenly began speaking to Beth. She reported that it was swearing at her, calling her names and telling her it would never leave and that she couldn't force it to go. Our first attempt to expel it met with only partial success, so I urged Beth to call in Archangel Michael to facilitate the removal. With his help, this hostile being was removed and escorted on to a new destination. We then thanked Archangel Michael for his service, and he departed.

After this encounter, Beth revealed that in the past week, another voice had surfaced. This voice told her, "You steal people's souls with your eyes when you look at them." I asked if she thought this was true—that she stole people's souls with her eyes. She replied that she didn't know if it was true or not. I explained that this was not the kind of thing a person would say to herself, nor did I think it was likely she was stealing souls with a glance. It was obvious to me that the voice was an entity, but not to Beth. This is an example of how an entity can strongly influence someone.

We directed our attention to this new creature, which neither Beth nor her mother could detect. I was able to perceive it in my body as canine-like energy, and I remarked to them that I felt what I termed "wolf energy." Beth's mother said, "Oh, yes. I feel that!" We then addressed our inquiries to "wolf energy," and the entity responded. It told Beth that it was certainly not an entity—that it was an aspect of her personality. I had a strong intuition that this entity was picking up on the "wolf medicine" Beth carried and was attempting to cloak itself in it to deceive us. I shared this with her and said I was sure this creature was an entity.

When the entity heard me say that, it switched tactics and told Beth that it had been with her for a very long time and that it would never leave. I asked her if she wanted to expel this creature, and she vigorously replied that she did. We continued the process, and she removed the entity with the higher guides' assistance and sent it off with them, feeling empowered by her act. We then asked Archangel Michael to fill the spaces vacated by these energies.

I explained to Beth and her mother everything I knew about entities and their capacities for deception. Beth said she now understood more clearly what these beings were and how they behaved, and vowed to be more careful in the future. I encouraged her to enact the entity removal process whenever she suspected the presence of one, especially if it involved internal voices. There is no harm in doing the process, I added, and if there is zero response, it is most likely something else that is causing your symptoms.

Beth said she had noticed several more tears in her aura in the weeks between visits and was concerned about them. I replied that I felt it was the entity we had just removed that had caused those tears. Again, I handed her my crystal tool from the altar and directed her to sew them up, which she expertly did. I then gave her more extensive guidance on protecting her aura and advised her to remember to ask her guides for help whenever she had questions. She replied that she was now much more aware of her aura and would be more diligent in caring for herself and her energy field. I told her I was glad to hear about her new attitude toward self-care.

Following this, I asked Beth to prepare for the shamanic journey. I made room next to the altar and spread out a pad for her to lie on. As she relaxed more deeply, I darkened the room and then led her down the steps into the unconscious. When she called for a higher guide, she excitedly reported that a large wolf had appeared before her. After confirming that he was the appropriate guide for the journey, I suggested that Beth ask Wolf to proceed with more healing. When she did, he transported her to a scene in which there were several boxes. I advised her to ask Wolf to open the boxes, at which point he said we only needed to open one. When he opened it, Beth said she found there was "a small self, inside." I explained that this was another soul fragment that she could bring back into herself via her heart or solar plexus. She reported that the fragment readily came back into her heart and reintegrated smoothly.

After pausing for a few moments, Wolf then took Beth to what she described as a deep well. She could see that there was another fragment of herself in the well, and when she asked Wolf to help, he brought this piece up from the depths. I asked if she could bring this fragment back in, and she replied with concern that it didn't want to come back into her. I suggested she ask Wolf for more information about the soul piece, and he revealed that it was a teenage part that was very rebellious and angry at her. I explained that this was common with teenage fragments and that we first needed to inform it of Beth's present situation.

I then guided Beth in a long conversation with the soul piece as she explained to it all that had happened since it had split off. She ended her story by describing who she had become up to the present moment and added that she very much wanted this piece of herself to return. I suggested also promising this fragment that she would care for it and would not do anything to cause it to split off again. Beth gave her pledge and, after a long pause, the piece agreed to come back. Beth was able to reincorporate it into her solar plexus and reported that she could feel it merge smoothly back into herself. We were all relieved that she had recovered this lively and integral fragment.

Wolf then transported Beth on to the next soul piece. This very young part was also hesitant to rejoin her, so I again guided Beth in another lengthy discussion that allowed the fragment to feel safe about returning. Finally, it elected to rejoin her, and she reported that it had entered her heart chakra and seamlessly assimilated.

When Beth had completed the retrieval, Wolf brought in a final fragment that quickly and eagerly went back into her heart center and reconnected. When she finished, she remarked that she felt much more stable and whole with all these soul pieces back inside herself. I commended her on her willingness to accept these lost fragments, reincorporate them and ensure their safety.

I then suggested that Beth ask if there were any past-life issues on which we could work. Wolf said there was one and immediately transported her into the past life. He presented her with an overview of that lifetime and explained that it involved a "complex of issues involving racism and discrimination." I asked her if she wanted to heal the energetic deposit that she carried from these past-life issues, and she replied that she did. I then prompted her to ask Wolf if he could transmute and clear the entire complex, from both the past life and from this one. He responded that he would clear most of it but that "some has to remain for now." Beth requested that he clear what he could, which he immediately did.

Wolf explained to Beth that the entities had been using these archived energies as ammunition to berate her as racist. She was susceptible to this due to the energetic deposits of her past-life racist actions—she believed the accusing voices because there was some truth to their words. As Beth accepted and integrated what Wolf told her, he cleared another portion of those deposits. I encouraged her to be as open as possible and incorporate all the information she could at this time; this process continued for several minutes.

As Beth completed that task, I urged her to ask if she had been actively calling in entities. Wolf answered that she had indeed been doing this. We asked for more clarity about this and whether he could heal it. Wolf gave her a detailed explanation of how and why she was inviting these entities; he said he could clear this, but that it would take some time. Beth requested that Wolf proceed with this healing in whatever manner was appropriate. He assured her that he would do all he could to fulfill her request.

Once Wolf completed his work, he advised Beth that we had done enough for the day. I prompted her to ask him to return her to the gateway, and she was instantly there. They conversed for a while, as she thanked Wolf for helping her and agreed to continue working together. I brought her back up into our everyday reality and gave her time to adjust back into the healing room.

When Beth was able to sit up, she remarked that she now felt much more whole, more comfortable in her own skin and filled with some shining new energies. She was happily glowing and smiling as I encouraged her to continue working with Wolf, using the shamanic journey format. In case she needed more help navigating the journey, I suggested that her skillful mother, who had witnessed the sessions, would be able to help guide her. Her mother smiled and immediately agreed, and they both eagerly vowed to continue the work.

I then inquired about the sacred altar that I had suggested Beth create after our last session. She replied that she had not gotten around to it yet, but was definitely planning to do it. I again recommended that she establish and use her sacred altar as the focal point for working with her guides. I also explained the importance of daily grounding her body and energy field into Mother Earth and assured her that this would promote her stability and balance. I urged her to keep her aura pulled in close to her body as a way to minimize intrusions, rather than letting it extend into her environment where it would be more permeable to others. She agreed that this was important and promised she would try to remember it. Beth also announced that she was committed to caring for herself now, which we were delighted to hear.

I asked Beth and her mother what they planned to do about Beth's psychiatrist, now that all her symptoms were gone. They both agreed that she no longer needed to see him or take the medications, but they were unsure how to proceed. I told them it was necessary to work with the doctor to wean Beth off of the intense psychoactive drugs she had been taking, which could take some time. Beth said she felt confident that she now had tools and techniques to use to do more healing and repair work on herself. She also had a greater understanding of the spiritual realm, the beings in it, and how to work with them. I told her she was always welcome to come back at any time if she felt she needed my help.

Beth then expressed her gratitude to me for guiding her through such an extensive healing process, and I told her that it was my pleasure to help her. We ended our session by thanking all our guides and closing sacred space. Beth's appearance had again changed markedly during this second session. I noticed that she was now a radiant, calm, self-assured and happy young woman. I thanked our guides silently for this powerful transformation.

Beth continued to do well and, several years later, her mother told me that Beth had made steady improvement by working with all her guides. The big news was that she had gotten married and was expecting a baby. Beth had shown everyone in her family that she was feeling healthy, whole and happy in her life. Her mother and I were, of course, both thrilled.

* * *

Guided Shamanic Journey Process

Overview:

Mastering some form of progressive relaxation, visualization or hypnotic induction technique is very helpful for gently guiding the client into an altered state. There are a great many books on shamanic practice that can provide a cognitive understanding, as well as an ever-increasing number of shamanic offerings online. One's direct experience with nonphysical realities and spirit guides, gained by actually applying the information presented here, will be the best teacher. We learn by doing and exploring.

As always, begin by opening sacred space and creating a suitable energetic container for this process. I offer my clients the option to lie down on a pad with a blanket and pillow or sit up for the journey. The person must be comfortable, feel safe and not be distracted. I recommend using an eye mask to minimize external disturbances and to facilitate better visions. Be sure to advise anyone you work with that they will need to communicate aloud with you throughout the process. I recommend recording the entire session so that the client can listen to it again and again.

For the induction, I use a very simple guided relaxation process in which I ask the client to imagine, as vividly as possible, the scenes I describe. Relaxation is essential, as is trust in the practitioner. On the descending and ascending of the stairs, I generally use 10 steps as a good number of footfalls for most people. Describe to them what they are feeling as they reach each level—for example, "You feel your body growing heavier as you step down." The descent speed can vary depending upon the person, but it should be gradual, steady and relaxed. I suggest writing out a script of everything you plan to say; follow it until you have mastered a fluid presentation.

I recommend using spirit guides who are "of the light." Direct the person to ask three separate times if the being who appears to them is of the light. I work only with guides who reply with a strong "yes" all three times. I was taught, and my experience confirms, that a spirit being cannot lie three times in a row. Beings who are not of the light can be ambiguous or murky, ineffectual, poor communicators, merely curious, or of malevolent intent—none of which will give you optimal results. If you doubt the spirit's integrity, it's best to send it away and have the client call again until you are satisfied and feel confident about a guide's motivations and integrity.

Ask for the guide's name, if not already known, for ease of communication and to build the client's relationship with this helper spirit. If the person cannot communicate clearly with the guide, the higher being can frequently augment the client's perception if they request it. However, if the person cannot perceive and communicate distinctly with a helping spirit, they will not be able to participate fully in this shamanic process and it is usually not fruitful for them to continue with the guided journey as outlined. If that is the case, any meditation and guided imagery techniques, or hypnotherapy methods you have mastered, may be used to address their issues. A very small percentage of clients are in this category.

When I first began doing this type of energy work, I facilitated my clients' travels into shamanic altered states but did not actively guide them after delivering them to the "lower world." I outlined what they needed to do once they arrived in the lower realms and assumed that they would be able to accomplish it by themselves. I soon realized that this did not work well for most people. Clients could not navigate the non-ordinary realities effectively by themselves—even with their guides; furthermore, they were not able to generate the questions needed to interact with their helping spirits. Even clients experienced in shamanic journeying did not do well. For this reason, I began to orchestrate the process and discovered that the guided method presented here produced far superior results. After a while, I opted to begin with the much simpler progressive relaxation and visualization technique I now use because it delivers the client more directly and effectively to an experiential non-ordinary reality.

Spirit guides can provide direction, answer questions and perform energetic clearing, repair and healing if they are requested to do so by the client. Higher beings are generally not permitted to do any of this on their own because humans have free will, and all ethical spirit beings will respect this. This is the reason the individual must state to the guide that they desire and request specific actions. Likewise, the practitioner must also honor the free will and desires of the client.

The practitioner should be familiar with and able to navigate the nonphysical realms of consciousness into which they guide the client. Additionally, having a seasoned practitioner accompany the journeyer instills trust and promotes a deeper and smoother journey. Before starting the journey process, the facilitator must have a general itinerary in mind. This list includes all issues and conditions discussed in the intake interview with the client in addition to potential interventions such as cord removal, soul retrieval, past-life archives and ancestor work (as time permits and as directed by the spirit guide).

It is equally essential for the practitioner to be open to intuition, feelings, experience, and information from the spirit realm. There are always many options in the multiverse and many decisions to be made. If you, as the facilitator, get stuck, hit a dead end, or are uncertain what to do, you can always ask the guide for help.

The spirit helper will usually tell the person when each section is complete and when the journey itself needs to end. The higher being can then deliver the client to the gateway where the journey began and from there, you can guide them back up the stairs. Again, this ascent is slow, and the facilitator should describe each step for them, such as: "Step three. You are feeling much lighter and more whole." You can remind them of specifics of the journey to help them remember salient points, especially if they have pledged to take a particular action or have been given other assignments by their guide.

Once the client is back in the everyday realm, give them time to adjust, reflect, ask questions or take notes. If the healing work involved significant removal of archived energy, the practitioner should fill the client's aura with uplifting energy to replace it. Alternatively, you can instruct the client to request that the higher guide do this at the close of the journey. Once complete, end your session by closing sacred space and thanking the spirit helpers who assisted. When the individual is ready to depart, ensure they feel safe, competent, balanced and grounded before allowing them to go out into the world.

Step-by-Step Process:

1. Begin by giving the client an overview of the process that allows them to feel safe, relaxed and ready to proceed.
2. Use an induction technique including progressive relaxation, guided visualization, deep breathing and release of all tension, thoughts, ideas and expectations to promote a fluid entry into an altered state.

3. Once the client is very relaxed and breathing slowly, have them imagine standing at the top of a flight of 10 steps leading down into their unconscious.

4. Ask the client if they can perceive these steps. If so, begin walking them down. If not, have them imagine the steps as vividly as possible and then start the descent. Be sure to describe each step as they reach it, counting down slowly from 10 to 1.

5. At the bottom step, tell the client they have reached the bottom of the stairs and that a path stretches out before them. Ask if they can perceive this path. If so, proceed; if not, ask them to imagine the path—as clearly as they can—extending before them.

6. Direct them to walk along the path until they reach a stone gateway (or another portal, if you prefer) and request that they let you know when they have walked through it.

   The client is now in a light trance state in a nonphysical reality and ready to start the journey. Make sure they can describe to you what they are experiencing throughout the session. This capacity to narrate experiences varies considerably with each individual, yet all can usually communicate clearly enough with proper guidance.

7. Ask the journeyer to call in a higher guide and to let you know who comes in to be with them. This normally takes less than a minute.

   Determine whether it is an appropriate helping spirit for the work you want to do, and ensure that the being is of the light, as described earlier. Frequently, the client asks me how to call in a guide. I tell them to state aloud: "I call in a higher guide." Sometimes the first being to appear is an overseer, especially if it is an archangel or a religious figure. They will tell you this if you ask, and will be able to send in an appropriate spirit being to assist with the actual process. Occasionally, a deceased ancestor comes in. Most often, this being is there for support rather than being the actual guide. They will also tell you this if you ask.

8. Once the client establishes a good connection with the guide, the practitioner directs the client's interactions with that spirit being throughout the session.

   Begin by having the individual ask the guide to take them to the source of each condition they have discussed with you. Alternatively, you could suggest that they ask their guide questions regarding soul retrieval, past lives, ancestor work or any other topic that you think could be beneficial for them to explore. The journey will unfold from there.

9. Proceed from issue to issue until the spirit being lets you know that the journey is complete. At that point, have the client request the guide return them to the gateway. The person can then thank their guide and discuss any further work that they might accomplish together.

10. When the client is ready, bring them slowly up the steps, counting from one to ten, until they are back at the top of the stairs. Then help them gently return to our everyday reality, and give them time to adjust and integrate their experiences.

Cord Removal Process

Overview:

The first case study with Beth included a description of the removal of cording. What are cords? This term refers to etheric, parasitic connections that commonly form between people. Cords can also connect people to places, objects, past events or trauma. Most people can perceive (see, feel, sense, imagine) these cords when they are in an altered state and often describe them as long, stringy ropes, vines or wires. These can appear singular or multiple, thin or thick, single- or multi-stranded, and long or short. These cords are always a conduit for draining energy from someone. They can be used to send or receive feelings of pain, guilt, fear, anger and control, and can even cause a person to obsess about something without knowing why.

Cords are formed unconsciously and are very common between family members, partners and those who are in other close relationships. The healthy connections, such as love and trust that exist between people are not cords. We are all inextricably linked, connected to everything in the Universe; these beneficial connections are sacred and cannot be broken. Cords are exclusively detrimental connections that are not healthy for either individual.

I usually facilitate the cord removal process within the shamanic journey where the client is already in an altered state with the spirit helper present. The guides know if there is cording, who it is with and if we can address it. If the journeyer has cords with more than one person, the guide will know which person should appear first. It doesn't matter whether the cords are with incarnated individuals or the deceased, since everyone will appear in an etheric body. Occasionally, the spirit guide will say that there are additional people with whom the client has cords, but advises that now is not the time to remove them.

I always direct clients to remove every part of each cord instead of cutting it because, in cutting it, the connections remain in both people. Some clients insist they had already cut a specific cord when their guide brings in a person with whom the cord is still intact. Perhaps the cords regrew because they were not completely removed, or there may have been continued adverse effects from the attachment itself.

If the person with whom there is cording is threatening, scary or abusive to your client, take extra precautions. The client can either ask their guide for protection or call in the other person's guide and request that they protect everyone involved.

Cord removal results in a significant freeing of an individual's energy and volition, along with an increased sense of well-being. The client's relationship with the other person—whether living or deceased—can improve appreciably, since all the healthy connections remain. Once someone accomplishes this process during their journey, they most likely can perform it again without your guidance if the need arises. I generally ask my clients if they feel capable of accomplishing future cord removal, especially if the guide has indicated they have cording with more people.

Step-by-Step Process:

1. Direct the client to ask their spirit helper if there is cording that can be removed. If so, have them ask the guide to bring that person into their presence (this will be in an etheric body).

2. Ask the client if they can perceive this person and the cords that exist between them. Nearly everyone can perceive both; if they cannot perceive the cords, have the client vividly imagine them. Alternatively, the client can ask their guide to augment their perception to enhance the experience, or ask the guide to remove and transmute the cords.

3. Direct the client to first remove the cords from their own body, with loving-kindness for the learning they received from the cording. Cords frequently have many little rootlets or tendrils in the body. If this is the case, instruct the client to carefully remove each one of these tendrils. We do this with loving-kindness to avoid generating karma.

4. Once the client's side of the cording is detached, direct them to ask the other person if they would like the cord(s) removed from their body.

   If the reply is no, I suggest having the client request that their guide explain to the person why it would benefit them to have the cord removed. This usually results in the person then saying yes. If the answer is yes, the client removes the cording from the other person, with loving-kindness, in the same manner as before.

5. Once the cord is completely removed from both parties, ask the client to coil it like a rope. Have them visualize a burning bowl nearby, and instruct them to place the cord into the burning bowl.

6. Direct the client to call in the violet flame of transmutation, which consumes the cord and transmutes it into light.

   Most clients report seeing the flame, but if not, ask them to imagine it vividly. They can also use this light to cleanse and heal any wounds that remain from the cording if they choose. If the client wishes to speak to the other person for any reason, let them know that this is their opportunity to do it. Then, you can allow the other person speak, if they so choose.

7. When finished, the client asks the guide to take the other person back to where they belong.

8. Direct your client to ask if there are more people with whom they have cording to remove. If there are, proceed in the same manner with each new person until the guide indicates the entire process is complete. The practitioner then moves the client along to the next healing topic.

Chapter 10

Soul Retrieval

Sandra Ingerman, a well-known authority on soul retrievals, defines *soul* as "our essence, life force, the part of our vitality that keeps us alive and thriving."[8] This definition is important since, for many people, *soul* is a nebulous word without clear meaning. In her book *Soul Retrieval*, Sandra also describes *soul loss* as "a spiritual illness that causes emotional and physical disease."[9] This illness results from "losing crucial parts of ourselves that provide us with life and vitality."[10] It is not the loss of an actual piece of the soul but the loss of a vital part of oneself, sometimes experienced as light or awareness, that leaves the person without health, vitality or a sense of wholeness.

This type of loss is quite common in our modern culture, and many people with whom I have worked have experienced it at least once. Any situation or experience in life that is beyond a person's capacity to contain will split off as a fragment of that person. The trauma can be mental, emotional, psychological, physical or even spiritual.

Soul retrieval refers to the ancient shamanic practice of bringing back these vital pieces which have been "lost" or split off by life experiences. Traditionally, soul retrieval is performed for an individual by a shaman or other practitioner, who can enter into other realities or spiritual realms to locate, collect and return with the missing piece. Once this missing soul fragment is retrieved, the shaman uses their breath to direct it back into the person to whom it belongs. This classical practice has been used for countless millennia by many traditional cultures, which consider soul loss a common cause of illness. The retrieval and reintegration of the lost pieces cures the illness and restores the person's wellness.

The soul piece that cleaves off carries with it both the energetic charge and the memory of the traumatic experience. Many fragments may also contain other vital aspects of the individual, such as abilities and gifts. For example, a piece could hold musical or artistic talents that the person remembers having had earlier in life but have since disappeared. It is necessary to seek out, retrieve and reinstate these fragments because they rarely come back on their own. The piece that splits off resides in a nonphysical dimension, in suspended animation, until someone comes to collect it and return it home.

The type of shock that causes a split can be as varied as a sudden fright, surgery, an accident, war, terrorism, natural disasters, abuse or injury, or loss of a family member, a friend or even a pet. In other words, any event that is traumatic to the person can precipitate fragmentation. This splitting off is a survival mechanism that allows the individual to survive an experience that would otherwise be too much to endure. The process is called *dissociation* by psychologists. This soul loss is not as extreme as dissociative identity disorder (D.I.D.) since the splits are small fragments of the self rather than distinct personality states. Many people also have what are referred to in the Internal Family Systems psychotherapy model as "parts." These are also dissociated aspects of the person that are usually residing within the body of the individual, as opposed to fragments that have been externalized. It is my experience that, when encountered, these "parts" can also be reintegrated back into the larger Self by the appropriate spirit helper.

Because the soul piece that splits off carries the entire energetic charge and memory of the event, a person may have little or no memory of the incident that caused the fragmentation. I believe a vast majority of people are missing a piece of themselves and do not know it. An individual may sense that something is wrong and may not feel completely whole but not understand what has happened or how to remedy it. The fact that soul loss is not recognized as an ailment in our culture adds to the lack of awareness of this widespread condition. Some common signs that someone has lost soul pieces are depression, a feeling of being broken or missing a part, insomnia, fear or anxiety, and the loss of memories or episodes of one's life.

The soul retrieval method presented here does not require a shaman skilled in searching non-ordinary realities to find and retrieve the lost fragment. Any conscientious practitioner will be able to facilitate the process. The client participates in finding and reincorporating their own soul pieces and is further healed by the return of their memories. They can see the conditions under which the piece split off, understand why and how it separated, and then have the opportunity to facilitate the fragment's return.

Because the individual immediately identifies with the soul piece and has the memory associated with it return, they can fully connect with and reintegrate it immediately. Clients retain a clear memory of the entire process upon their return to ordinary reality and are empowered by participating in the retrieval. The case studies described throughout this book present varied examples of soul retrievals. I recommend giving the client a simple explanation of the retrieval process before embarking on the shamanic journey to clarify the experience.

Again, the higher guides know everything about a person, including all events in this and all other incarnations. Thus, they know where all fragments are, the order in which to retrieve them and the best method for rejoining them to the person. Guides can also facilitate soul retrievals for any past lives that need healing. Soul retrievals done in this way have built-in safeguards, since the higher guides will not do work that is not permitted and will advise the client if there is some reason the fragment cannot be returned.

Soul retrievals for ancestors, families and tribes, or other groups of people may be enacted by connecting with the appropriate guide. We are multidimensional beings simultaneously inhabiting expanded group bodies in the transpersonal realms. I believe there are spirit guides who work with these collective bodies and that this represents an exciting topic for future research.

* * *

Amanda, a fellow healing practitioner whom I had known for many years, contacted me to ask about working on three specific things. Her issues included the feeling of not belonging, the fear of being in bodily pain and her inability to relax deeply or to trust. These were lifelong conditions, and none of the considerable work she had previously done on herself had impacted them. She wanted new insights and solutions, and wondered if the work I did could help her. I responded that I was sure that we could gain valuable insights from her participation in a guided shamanic journey.

As I greeted Amanda, I noticed that her short brown hair had highlights of blond and green and that she was in her usual cheery mood. We settled into my healing room, opened sacred space and called in our spiritual support. I began with the rounds of energy cleansings of her aura and then guided her to extract impeding energies from within her body with my black tourmaline. She told me she was surprised about the process of using a stone to extract energy and found it very powerful.

Hearing this, I gave her a stone from my altar to use as her personal extraction stone. Amanda was thrilled to have the stone, and I led her through a process of connecting to it. First, I encouraged her to ask the stone its name, and being a new experience for her, she was surprised and delighted to hear a clear answer from the stone. I then described how she could use it at home to do the same type of extraction she had just done. I reviewed the process again in detail and jotted down a few notes for her.

Following that, I seated Amanda in front of my altar and explained we would be looking for any entities that she might be carrying. As I guided her in the entity removal process, she located and expelled several non-troublesome beings and requested that the guides take them safely away. As she removed each creature, she remarked that she felt lighter, as if heavy layers were being peeled off of her, one by one.

Next, I gave Amanda an overview of the shamanic journey, which she was very eager to experience. After making sure she was comfortable on a pad alongside the altar, I brought her down the steps into the unconscious. She signaled me when she had passed through the gateway, and I directed her to call in a higher guide. Within moments, a beautiful, shining woman dressed in a fancy, flowing gown appeared. Amanda was very impressed by her appearance and gave me a vivid description of her.

I then instructed Amanda to ask this being if she was of the light, to which the startling answer was "no." Amanda was disappointed, so I mentioned that this frequently happens and suggested she call in her master-healer guide. Having made this request, she reported that an enormous being appeared who, when questioned, replied, "I am the light."

I directed Amanda to ask the luminous guide to take her to the source of her feeling of not belonging. With surprise, she reported that she was looking at herself as a baby, standing up in her crib. Her mother and father were present in the same room, not far away, but they were singularly preoccupied with their own activities. Neither had the slightest interest or desire to interact with her in any way. Amanda confided that this experience was "emotionally crushing" for both her infant and adult selves and, as she witnessed this scene, she began to cry freely.

Amanda then reported that her master healer wanted me to cleanse all the painful, crushing energy sequestered in her body as a result of her parents' behavior. I agreed but first gave her a small ceremonial doll from my altar and told her to place it over her heart. I explained that the doll would collect and heal the toxic programming that this and similar events had instilled in her. I also instructed her to envision the doll filling the space where the pain had been with vibrant and loving energy.

When she was ready, I blew cleansing aromatic waters over her aura and began to rattle vigorously in a counter-clockwise circle just above her body. The percussion of my Amazonian rattle served to break up the concretized noxious energies. I then removed them from her field and sent them into my altar ground. When finished, I checked to see if Amanda had completed her work with the doll, and she said it had been "a magic experience" for her. I told her I was glad to hear it as I collected and cleansed the doll before returning it to my altar.

I then suggested that Amanda request her guide to put a shield of protection around her that would prevent any disabling and obstructing energies from coming into her body and energy field. She reported that he had fulfilled this request at once, and she could feel a luminous envelope surrounding her. The master healer asked me to rattle again and blow additional aromatic waters over her aura and physical body. He indicated that this was to remove the damage caused by her parents' chronic neglect of her needs throughout her childhood. I did as he requested, cleansing the last of the repulsive energies from her, and then we paused to let these experiences assimilate.

Next, I told Amanda to ask if she had soul fragments that we could retrieve at this time. The light being replied that there were many, and Amanda immediately said she could see them. They appeared "like a constellation of stars in the sky," and there were too many to count. I suggested she ask if the higher guide could bring them back as a group since there were so many. His answer was, "Certainly," as he gathered them up in a cluster and brought them back to Amanda. I instructed her to put them all into her body, either through her heart or solar plexus chakras, and to let them reintegrate back into her.

I then explained these were all pieces of herself, which had split off over time through trauma of one kind or another. "Yes, I can feel that," she said as she finished installing them. I counseled her on caring for the fragments, stressing that it was vital for them to stay and reincorporate into her larger self. She promised to make this a daily priority.

Since Amanda had a healing practice of her own, she had many questions, both for me and her guide, about doing energy healing work on others. Her master healer imparted some basic instructions for approaching energy work, and I told her that she and I would discuss it in more detail after the journey. He then stressed that most of all, Amanda needed to take her time and not hurry things. He told her new healing tools for working on others would be coming to her and repeated that she should be patient and allow these tools to arrive. "Do not go out and buy them," he added with emphasis. He also counseled her to let her process for doing energy work come to her over time. "Don't go out looking for it!" he cautioned. "It will come to you." *Wise words for all of us,* I thought, and told her I agreed with her guide.

Continuing the journey, we asked about Amanda's fear of pain. The master healer took her to a scene where she saw her six-year-old self in acute pain. She had fallen, dislocating her knee and lay in pain and fear for hours before anyone came to help her. We asked how to clear the archived trauma of this event, and the guide again requested that I use medicinal waters and rattle over her knee. As soon as I completed this, he instructed me to suck black, sticky energy out of her third eye and crown chakras using a crystal from my altar, which I promptly did.

Amanda reported that each of these actions was significant in removing trapped pockets of pain and fear from her body. Then, to finish the process, the spirit being asked me to cleanse her entire energy field once more. When I finished, I asked Amanda how she felt, and she replied, "I feel refreshed and renewed." I told her I was delighted she felt so much better and had successfully removed the disruptive energies.

Her guide then informed us that we had done enough work for one session. I told Amanda to ask to return to the gateway where she had begun the journey. Once there, I reminded her to thank him for the remarkable work he had done and to ask if she could work directly with him in the future. He replied that he was her master-healer guide and would be available to her whenever she wanted to work on healing. She thanked him again and said she was very excited to have met him.

I brought Amanda back up the steps into our everyday reality and asked once more how she felt. She was smiling as she animatedly replied that she was tired but exhilarated from the extraordinary healing work we had accomplished. We talked for a long while, allowing her to recover from her journey, and then she scheduled another session to complete the issues we could not fit into this extensive session. We thanked our spiritual support and closed sacred space.

* * *

Soul Retrieval Process
Overview:

This process unfolds within the guided shamanic journey and is directed by the spirit guide and the practitioner. The guide may take the journeyer to the fragment or might bring it to the client. Request as much detail as possible from the person to clearly understand what is happening in the encounter.

Occasionally, the client doesn't completely understand what they are experiencing or lacks a clear perception of the fragment. If necessary, have them ask the spirit being for more clarity or information until both you and the journeyer understand the situation. The client can narrate their experience as they move through the process. Ask them to let you know when the retrieval is complete and how they feel once the fragment reintegrates. Even if you can journey shamanically with the client or clairvoyantly see what is happening, it is important to hear directly what they experience.

Soul pieces apparently need to be retrieved in a specific order and also require a particular timing. The guide may state that some fragments must remain for now and be collected later. There also seems to be an optimal number of retrievals per session for each person. The helping spirit will generally inform the journeyer about these parameters as part of the process. It is not unusual for clients to have many fragments or even clusters of them, and these can frequently be brought in as a group by the higher guide if specifically asked to do this.

If a fragment is unwilling to return, more communication is needed to educate it and bring it into the present time. The soul piece, residing in nonphysical reality in a state of suspended animation, is entirely unaware of the individual's life progression since it left. Survivors of sexual or physical abuse are likely to have reluctant fragments. This is because the pieces are unaware that the life situation of the person has changed. Soul pieces can be fearful or angry and, understandably, do not want to return to the same circumstances that caused the original split.

Substantial resistance can also occur with teenage fragments; they may be angry and rebellious, and even demean the person trying to retrieve them. A very young soul fragment may be unsure about returning because of chaotic or dangerous experiences, such as having a family member with a significant mental illness. Informing the fragment about what has happened in the person's life since it split off generally removes any hesitancy. The client can explain that they are now grown, no longer live at home and that the environment is safe for the fragment. I have yet to witness a soul piece refuse to return, although some do need quite a bit of coaxing.

Twice, I have had clients who did not want their soul pieces back, and in both cases, they were incest survivors. Neither wanted the fragment because it had the painful memories of the event that caused the split. One client emphatically stated, "I don't want all that horrible and scary stuff back." Nevertheless, it is crucial to reunite these lost pieces for the client to again be whole. The guide can assist the person in being able to understand, soften, heal or reframe the trauma. As a practitioner, experience with soul retrievals is helpful to troubleshoot and actively facilitate the dialogue between a fragment and your client.

Once a soul piece has been returned, the client needs to make accommodation for it. In other words, the person must be attentive to the needs and feelings of the returned fragment since it can split off again if it does not feel welcome. This accommodation might involve conversations with the restored aspects, engaging in activities that are fun for a younger self, re-parenting the fragment, being more playful in general, spending more time in nature and being less busy. The practitioner can recommend that the client be more mindful, present, creative, and very attuned to their emotions as the new piece completely integrates.

Step-by-Step Process:

1. Once the client is in the unconscious and connected with a light-filled spirit helper, begin by having them ask the guide if there are any lost fragments or missing pieces to be retrieved. If the answer is yes, the client asks to meet the first piece. Tell the person to let you know what they perceive and experience. If the answer is no, proceed on to another facet of the guided shamanic journey.

2. When the fragment is present, either the client or the guide will engage with the piece to ensure that it is ready to return. If it is, the client or the spirit being can collect the fragment and reinstate it into the body. I suggest bringing it back in through either the heart chakra or the solar plexus. If it does not want to return, that issue must be addressed and resolved before proceeding.

3. Ask the client to tell you when the reincorporation is complete, and then ask if there are more pieces to recover.

4. If there are, continue in the same manner until the guide says the retrieval process is finished. It is common for people to have multiple fragments. You can also have the client ask the soul piece or their guide if there are any specific actions or activities they might bring into their life to help each soul piece re-incorporate. Once there are no remaining pieces to retrieve at present, proceed to another stage of the journey process.

* * *

Amanda returned a few weeks later, looking calm and much more relaxed. She said she was still strongly feeling and integrating the work we had previously done. I asked about her soul fragments, and she replied that she had taken time every day to connect with the memories and feelings of those younger parts of herself, and she had enjoyed it immensely.

Eager to continue the work, she reminded me that she wanted to address her inability to relax fully or trust. Amanda then confided that she had a history of liver disease, on which she had been working for many years, and she had a few questions about it. She thought her liver was mostly healed but wanted to check on it in the journey and get direct input from her guide. I replied that we would most likely be able to accomplish these tasks.

Amanda and I began by opening sacred space and calling in our spiritual support. After completing the series of energy cleansings of her aura, I taught her how to carry these out for herself. When I seated her in front of my altar, she brought forth the extraction stone I had given her, and I guided her in using it to extract more layers of obstructing energy. Once she completed the task, she reported that more heavy, sticky energy left her body and entered the stone. She promptly discharged it into my altar ground and cleansed her stone with lavender floral water.

Checking for entities was our next step, and Amanda found several more that surfaced from her distant past. I assured her that this was common. I have observed that some entities appear to be embedded in layers or strata and only reveal themselves over time. With the guide's help, she expelled these creatures, clearing the way for further work.

Amanda then lay down beside the altar for the journey, and I led her down into the unconscious and through the gateway. She called for a higher guide and announced that a rather strange-looking being had presented himself. She questioned him, and he told her he was not of the light, so she sent him away and called again for a higher guide. The being who appeared this time declared he was of the light and that he was also the appropriate guide for the work we wanted to do. She described this spirit being in great detail, as his appearance was unique and very impressive. He also proved himself to be exceptionally eloquent, helpful and forthcoming throughout the journey, which was unusual for a guide.

I suggested that Amanda ask the spirit being if her liver was healthy. He answered that it was not and that he could extract the remaining toxic energy from it. I encouraged her to ask him to do this now, and he replied, "Absolutely!" She then reported that he gently placed his etheric hands, which had very long slender fingers, into her liver. He slowly began pulling out what she described as small stones and pieces of damaged tissue. This operation took only a short while and, when finished, he smoothed over her liver with his hands, healing and sealing it all.

He then announced that Amanda's liver was completely healed and, surprisingly, added an admonition to her not to be so critical of herself. He lovingly advised her to be gentle with herself and to take time to allow this healing to continue to unfold in her physical reality. He then underscored that she should always honor her body. Knowing Amanda, I felt this advice really hit the mark and told her so. She replied that she got the point and would be making some significant changes in her behavior.

I then prompted Amanda to ask about clearing additional archived energy connected with her early childhood. The guide immediately presented her with a vision of her two- or three-year-old self, and she said it was like watching a movie. She saw herself as a joyous child, filled with light and curiosity, trusting and open to all—and she was broadly smiling as she said this. The higher being then proceeded to show her that, over time, the happy child had become coated with layers of conditioning that entirely covered up her innocent self. Amanda was extremely sad to witness this painful process and was nearly in tears as she did.

The spirit guide told Amanda that he wanted "to remove the encasing crust" which covered the young Amanda. I asked her how she felt about having the crust removed, and she replied that she felt some fear about doing that. When I asked why she was afraid, she replied that she wouldn't know who she was if the layers were gone. I then explained that these layers of encrustation were a consequence of the conditioning and programming she had received as a child. They constituted part of the false self, which had been covering up the real Amanda. "The casing has never really been you," I added, and her guide chimed in to confirm what I was saying.

Amanda decided she was ready for the crust removal and requested her guide to proceed. She reported that he very gently and carefully peeled off the accumulated layers, one by one, until she was revealed to herself as a "shiny new, yet original and sparkling self." Amanda said the feeling of having the encrusting layers removed was pure bliss and that now she was her authentic, pristine self.

The higher guide explained that being buried under the brittle coating had prevented Amanda from relaxing or trusting. She said she finally felt whole, as if her true self had just been resurrected and reborn. Shortly after, Amanda confided that she was thoroughly awed by the experience and the exhilaration she was experiencing now that she was free. I felt a wave of gratitude and joy wash over me as I heard her words, and I told her it was exciting to me, too.

Next, I suggested Amanda ask if she had any more soul fragments to be retrieved. Her guide replied, "No, you are whole," adding that all she needed was to step into her new self. When she asked how she could do that, he advised her to trust herself and her life. Amanda felt that this was not easy to do. The spirit being then showed her that she had a lot of fear energy swirling around inside and outside her body. He explained that the way through this fear was to have a deep trust in herself. Without the encasing conditioning, he said, she would now be able to respond to whatever arose and therefore did not need to live in fear of the unknown.

I interpreted this to mean that Amanda could focus on spending more time in the present moment. When I mentioned this to her, the guide concurred, saying that being present was the key. He then told her that her life is perfectly all right, just as it is—even if it doesn't look that way. "Trust," he insisted, "and be gentle with yourself, and you will jell." She deeply understood this counsel and pledged aloud that she would do it.

After this decree, I asked Amanda how she was feeling, and she replied that she felt fresh, clean, relaxed and well-nourished. The higher guide quickly reminded her to pay attention to all of her feelings and specifically told her to remember how she felt when I had given her the extraction stone at her previous visit. She recounted her feelings of delight and gratitude at the gift, which he encouraged, saying, "Feelings are in the body. Be in the body!" She confirmed that she was definitely getting the message and would make her best effort to comply.

After a few moments, Amanda told me that her guide advised her to cleanse her energy field with *palo santo* smoke daily, or as often as she remembered to do it. I asked if she had any of the aromatic wood at home, and she said she did. Next, her spirit being recommended taking some time to get to know her new heart-shaped stone, which was another stone from my altar that I had given to her. He gave her detailed instructions on using this stone to do energy work on herself; he also underscored that it was a personal tool for her, and she was not to use it on other people. After a pause, she added that he also gave her a list of recommended actions she could take daily to improve and maintain her health, which she found very helpful.

Amanda then expressed her gratitude to her guide for all of his assistance. He assured her he would always be available to her for any work she wished to do and urged her not to forget to call on him. She was thrilled when he added, "I want to work with you!" We were both tickled by such an unusual disclosure coming from a guide. I observed that he was truly unique and that she was fortunate to have such a proactive spirit guide. She readily agreed and said she was looking forward to calling upon him again soon.

At that point, the guide advised us we had completed our work for the day. Amanda requested that he return her to the gateway, and she was instantly there. She committed to calling on her helper spirit for further support and thanked him again for all he had done.

When Amanda was ready, I brought her back up the steps into the light of day. As she sat up and continued integrating the healing she had just experienced, I commented on how much softer and more alive she looked now after completing the journey. She laughed and replied that this was exactly how she felt, too. I congratulated her on achieving such intense and valuable healing, and told her to let me know how it all unfolded over the next few months. She promised she would stay in touch and expressed her gratitude to me for facilitating her journeys. We then closed our sacred space, thanking all our guides for their service.

Chapter 11

Childhood Trauma

CHILDHOOD TRAUMA IS EXTREMELY COMMON and, I believe, under-recognized in our modern Western culture. My focus here is on the trauma of family abuse and neglect rather than the collective damage from wars, disasters or displacement. There is ample evidence that trauma and abuse have been passed down in family systems for millennia. Added to this is the destabilization of both family and culture that occurs because of our collective trauma.

Childhood trauma is defined as any event a child experiences that is emotionally and/or physically painful or distressing. The event does not need to be severe or extreme to induce a disruptive response, as it is the child's perception of this event that matters. These could include incidents in which a child feels their life is—or might be—in danger. The trauma may be due to abuse or neglect, which the child might have experienced directly or witnessed others experiencing. This abuse can be physical, mental, emotional or psychological. Considerable research has been done on childhood trauma, much of which is decades old; however, a great deal of that research is still unintegrated into our present awareness and treatment modalities.

We know that childhood trauma has lasting mental, emotional and physical effects and can trigger both psychological and physical reactions that increase the risk of numerous health conditions. Psychiatrist Gabor Maté has stated that most physical, emotional and mental illness originates in coping patterns in response to infancy and childhood trauma. Having a history of trauma is a known risk factor for many adult diseases such as depression, post-traumatic stress disorder, most psychiatric disorders (especially addiction and Dissociative Identity Disorder) and physical illnesses such as cardiovascular disease, strokes, diabetes, cancer, autoimmune diseases and obesity. The direct biological effects from the extreme stress of trauma are well known and lead to a cascade of physiological reactions stemming from the release of stress hormones in the body. The release of these hormones causes inflammation that is a major risk factor for many adult diseases.

Not surprisingly, the risk of lasting mental and physical health problems increases with the number of adverse events a child has experienced, commonly referred to as a person's ACE score. The most common types of childhood trauma include physical, sexual and emotional abuse; physical or emotional neglect; witnessing domestic violence; living with substance abuse; living with family mental illness; incarceration of a family member; parental separation or divorce; the sudden death of a family member; and living with a family member who has an extreme or debilitating illness. This extensive list indicates that a great many people are carrying childhood trauma and suffering its effects. Nearly everyone I have worked with has endured some form of adverse childhood event, and that distress has led to chronic physical, mental or emotional dis-ease.

Individual archived trauma nearly always has its roots in the family and the lineage of that person. Lineage trauma and, by extension, its impact on society forms an additional layer that constitutes our collective or transpersonal trauma. This extensive distress affects every one of us at the societal level and has been largely ignored by medical science until recently. I hope that more research will focus on this crucial issue and that substantial collective healing will follow.

There have been extensive studies of overt and extreme trauma (some of which lasted many years), demonstrating that it results in significant mental and physical illness. The trauma of neglect is much less obvious but can result in psychological and physical dis-ease that greatly impairs a person's life. In these instances, it can be difficult for the person to realize that what they are experiencing could have been precipitated by childhood suffering. I have witnessed numerous cases in which a client has concluded that they must have a basic character flaw, are inherently defective or are somehow unworthy of better treatment—all of which are a child's normal reaction to distressing situations.

The child's survival mechanism may even have blocked the memory of the trauma, making it unlikely that the adult individual will be able to speak about it. And it is these cases of an unrecognized ordeal in which I nearly always see a vast improvement in a client's well-being in just one session of the shamanic journey. The following case study highlights the healing of childhood trauma.

* * *

Rose, a slender and sensitive woman, was a former shamanic studies student. She called one day to tell me she wanted to work with me on her lack of self-confidence. She knew this was a rather vague complaint, yet even though she was in her fifth decade, she was still plagued by the feeling that she couldn't function the way she wanted and that this held her back in life. I told her I was confident we would be able to discover what was blocking her, and we set an appointment for the following week.

It was good to see Rose again, and I had to admire her all-blue outfit with matching beret. After she settled in and relaxed in my healing room, I asked her to tell me more about her lack of self-confidence and inquired whether she had any specific memories related to this issue. In response, she gave me numerous examples and considerable background on her family of origin. Facing the altar, we opened sacred space and called in our spiritual support to begin the healing session.

First were the energy cleansings, and since Rose was attentive to keeping her field clean, there was only a small amount of dusky energy to remove. Next, I seated Rose in front of my altar, where we began searching for entities. In short order, she discovered four long-embedded entities blocking her access to a healthy sense of herself. She expelled each of these creatures in turn with the help of the guides. I then ensured she could perform the entity removal process to use if needed.

Rose was familiar with the shamanic journey work and was soon comfortably stretched out beside the altar, relaxed and ready to begin. I led her down the steps, through the gateway and directed her to call in a higher guide for the journey. At first, she reported that a small angel came in, and this angel then pointed toward a larger angel. When we questioned that angel, it was clear he was a light being and the appropriate guide for the journey. I advised her to ask him to take us to the trauma she had experienced at age 11.

At that age, Rose explained, her family had just moved from a spacious house with a beautiful large yard into a small, cramped building with no yard, which was located near a freeway. She remembered this as a devastating move because she was very connected to nature and greatly missed the yard in which she had grown up. We asked the guide to show her more of the circumstances around this period of her life, and he opened up a scene in which she witnessed the total dysfunction of her family dynamics.

Rose described her father as "an alcoholic workaholic" and her mother as "narcissistic and infantile." She observed herself trying to hold the family together by being the perfect daughter. Being perfect did not work and left her even more confused and overwhelmed by the family's dysfunctional behaviors. Rose had concluded it was her fault that the family would not come together and that this was because she was defective and a failure. Her higher guide gently and clearly explained that it was not her job to fix her family; the family issues were everyone's responsibility, not hers alone. She then acknowledged that she had made fixing the family her personal responsibility and now saw that it had never been the case.

I suggested the angel might be able to clear this archived trauma energy embedded inside Rose. She agreed and asked him to remove all the sticky darkness she could see she had accumulated. He replied that he would and immediately cleared the obscuring energy from both her adult and child bodies, at which point she smiled and remarked that she felt noticeably lighter.

I then encouraged Rose to ask if her guide could restore the original level of self-confidence she had had in her life. He replied that he could and would reinstate it, and we both felt a flood of confidence come into our awareness. Rose said she could actually feel her restored self-confidence as a physical sensation in her body and that it was breathtaking. I urged her to ask the angel to fill the space from which he had cleared the trauma with whatever qualities she wanted to manifest in her life. As she decreed aloud the attributes she desired, the guide added them to her energy field. When he finished, she shared her feelings of wonder as the uplifting energies came into her body. I replied that I, too, felt this potent energy movement within her.

The spirit being then transported Rose to a scene where she witnessed her older sister in the process of beating on her. We asked for the reason behind her sister's behavior, and he revealed that she was immersed fully in her own pain and trauma. Unsurprisingly, the sister likewise had no self-confidence and was adrift in her inner battles of torment and darkness. Rose realized that her sister had attempted to cope with her internal misery by projecting it all onto her little sister.

The revelation was that Rose could now see that this behavior was entirely about her sister and had nothing to do with her. Anyone in her position in the family would have received the same treatment from her sister. It was not personal and was not her fault. She told me that she could see the pain that her sister did not want to feel projected onto herself as a child as if it were a heavy, suffocating blanket.

I asked Rose if she wanted to remove this misplaced energy. She asked her guide to please clear all the projected torment and despair, which he instantly did. She then requested he replace those energies with new qualities and decreed her wishes aloud. A moment later, she reported that beautiful new vibrancy was flowing into her body, filling all the spaces where the darkness had been. When I asked how she felt, she told me she felt deeply healed and repaired and that all the pain of this event had disappeared.

Rose then remembered that she wanted to ask about a recurring dream she had had at that same age. In this dream, there was always a heavy iron chain around her neck. She wanted to know what this meant, as well as some of the other details she recalled. We asked the angel for clarity to understand her dream, and he showed her both the source and meaning of it. Although she did not share this information with me, Rose said she now thoroughly understood it but that the gloom and fear of the dream still remained. At my urging, she requested that the guide remove this dreadful energy and replace it with new vitality and a zest for life. When he completed this, she took a big breath and slowly released it with a sigh of contentment at the gratifying resolution of her dream.

The angel then showed Rose another scene of her 11-year-old self in which she had just finished writing a paper for a school assignment. Her mother had abruptly asked to read it, and Rose had dutifully handed it to her. Immediately after reading it, her mother began attacking her and telling her that her paper was terrible. With obvious distress, Rose explained that her mother had launched into a tirade about how poorly Rose had written it and how it reflected badly on her, the mother. Then, with rising anger, Rose reported that her mother began to completely re-write the paper there in front of her. Her mother did not ask her permission to do this, nor did she inquire about Rose's feelings in the matter, nor allow her to re-write it herself. Rose became increasingly upset as she witnessed this brutal betrayal and became even angrier as the scene impacted her fully.

I encouraged Rose to feel her intense emotions concerning this event and bring them into the present moment. We then engaged in a potent conversation about her mother's inappropriate behavior and the breach of trust this represented for young Rose. I suggested asking to see the larger context surrounding this event to understand it better. Rose observed that her mother was in significant distress about her own life because she considered it, up to that point, to be a dismal failure. She carried deep regrets about many of the life choices she had made and had never dealt with any of her grief. Rose said she could now see that her mother had always been trying to fulfill her own dreams through Rose's life, and it became painfully clear her mother was oblivious that her daughter was a separate person with her own life and feelings.

Rose shared that she had always known her mother was narcissistic, but now she understood the depth of her mother's self-absorption. More importantly, she understood her mother's treatment of her had nothing to do with her—it did not mean she was flawed, defective or unworthy of better treatment. Rose realized her feelings of being inept and ineffectual were part of her childhood coping mechanism and admitted always blaming herself for everything that went wrong in the family. She now recognized that over time this had become an ingrained habit. She added that she was stunned by the insight and clarity provided by her higher guide.

I told Rose I fully supported her new insights and encouraged her to ask the angel to clear out all of the misinterpreted events and misplaced habits that no longer served her. Rose made this request, and he immediately cleared them all. She then asked him to fill her with her unique dreams, joy, creativity and personal energy, which he instantly accomplished. When I asked how she felt, she described this experience as powerfully inspiring and likened it to a life-saving energy transfusion. We paused for a few minutes to allow it all to settle inside her.

I then mentioned my feeling that soul fragments had split off from Rose's younger self during her mother's attack on her and her school paper. She asked her guide if there were missing pieces from that event; he said there were and that we could retrieve them now. She instantly arrived at a scene where she could see a group of fragments related to that trauma. I suggested asking if the spirit helper could bring them in together rather than one by one. In response to her request, the angel scooped them all up and reinstated them into her body. I explained that it was her responsibility now to ensure that the fragments felt welcome and loved, which would prevent their splitting off again. Rose was thrilled to have these pieces back, understood their importance, and promised to care for them daily.

We then asked the spirit being about other archived trauma we could address, and he transported Rose to another episode in her life. She saw herself as a toddler happily playing in the yard not far from her father, who was sitting on the grass. She watched as her toddler-self crawled over to him and proceeded to climb up on his back. Both the toddler and adult Rose were shocked when her father shook her off and roughly pushed her away, leaving her in tears. "He had no space for me," she sobbed. The angel gently explained that this traumatic treatment she had endured as an innocent child caused her to believe that she could not trust any man.

I encouraged Rose to ask to see more of what lay behind her father's behavior. The spirit being disclosed that her father had pushed her away because of his unresolved pain and suffering. He had endured a very painful childhood, and Rose now understood this was the reason he had become an alcoholic. He could not face his own emotional and psychological wounding, she remarked at length. She mused about this for a few minutes and then proclaimed she was now able to receive this information about her father; she was able to accept him just as he had been, without any judgment. I congratulated her on this significant achievement and told her it was also critical to her own healing and self-acceptance.

I then suggested Rose might want to inquire about significant implications that her decision not to trust men has had on her life. She asked her guide to show her an overview of the life choices she had made, which he did in swift succession. As she took in these scenes, she realized she wanted to change her blanket distrust of all men since it did not serve her. I mentioned that her angelic guide could likely help her replace it with a healthy and discerning trust in men. She embraced this idea and requested he facilitate the exchange. Moments later, she reported that "the guide did some kind of rewiring in my body and mind" and that it felt remarkably beneficial.

Next, the spirit guide transported Rose to a scene of her older brother playing with her when she was a small child. She revealed that the older she got, the rougher the play until it eventually became him beating her up instead of playing with her. As a young child, she had looked up to her big brother and wanted to be with him, but because of his angry behavior, she ended up feeling abandoned by him.

Again, we asked her angel to disclose more of the story, and he revealed that her brother had long been struggling with Attention-Deficit/Hyperactivity Disorder. The guide explained that her brother's childhood trauma and repressed anger had caused the ADHD to manifest. On top of that, this diagnosis was a source of great shame to him and resulted in very low self-esteem. Rose then understood that her brother could not cope with his problems and the overall family dysfunction and saw her as an easy target for his anger.

Rose was very sad that this issue had driven them apart but realized she could not have done anything differently. She remembered that as they grew older, her brother was extremely jealous of her for being placed in classes for gifted students while he was not. Rose, in turn, had harbored great resentment toward him for many years because of his treatment of her. She then added that she was now reconsidering her feelings.

I encouraged Rose to ask to see exactly where her siblings' unhealthy habits had originated. She replied that her guide made it evident they had learned from their parents to deny, suppress and project their painful feelings—and she could see that everyone in the family was suffering from suppressed trauma and low self-esteem. No one was dealing with their emotional baggage, she observed, and "they were all projecting and attacking each other because they had no role models for any other kind of behavior." After a few moments, Rose confided that seeing it all with such clarity was a huge revelation. She now understood and accepted the truth of her family—and saw it objectively from an adult point of view.

Rose then asked the angel if there was any hope of her having a healthy relationship with her siblings in the present. He replied that, at this time, it was not possible because there was no means of having a relationship with a person who remained in total denial of their issues. Rose understood his answer but was tremendously sad to hear it. She sorrowfully told me that since her parents had both passed, she felt as if she had no family at all. I told her I, too, was sad about her family and encouraged her to journal her feelings to see what might emerge. She embraced this idea and said she would begin doing that right away.

At this point, the angel advised us that we had one final episode to review, which involved Rose's relationship with nature. He reminded Rose of how much she had loved spending time outdoors as a child—how it had fed her soul and how much she longed for it now. He also showed her why she had disconnected from nature: because of her family's move to an area with little access to the natural world, she had felt that nature was no longer there to help her. The higher being gently explained that this was entirely due to the family's unfortunate location and lack of connection to the environment and was not due to any fault or deficiency in nature.

Rose agreed it had been a child's reaction to pain and that nature had never betrayed her. I suggested she ask her guide to restore her lost childhood bond with the natural world. Rose immediately asked him to please repair her broken trust in nature, returning it to its pristine, vibrant condition. Moments later, she told me that "the guide did more rewiring on my brain," which she interpreted as the necessary repair and restoration. We paused for several minutes to let this experience integrate.

When I asked Rose how she felt after such an extensive journey, she said she was tired from all we had done but was excited and happy about everything that had happened. She was also thrilled with the incredible insights she now had. As we were getting ready to close, I recommended she ask if her angel could give her a gift of empowerment to help her in her daily life. She did, and he responded by pouring what she said appeared to be "star water" into her, filling her body and energy field with dazzling stars and light. Rose smiled broadly as she told me she now felt as if she was shiny, bright and glowing—and we both laughed with delight.

The guide then informed us that the journey was complete. I directed Rose to ask to return to the gateway, and instantly she was there. She thanked her angel for the incredible healing and wondrous gift she had received; he replied that he was always available to her and that she had only to call upon him. When they finished their conversation, I brought Rose back up the steps and into our everyday reality.

As I looked at her sitting beside my altar, I could see she was—without a doubt—shining. I mentioned this to her, and she replied that she could feel this new luminous energy in her aura and that it felt distinctly empowering. I congratulated her on the spectacular healing work she had accomplished, and we chatted for a while about her journey. I reminded Rose of her assignments of integrating her soul fragments, writing in her journal and reinforcing her new good habits daily. With a wide grin and sparkling eyes, she said she was now committed to her health. We both felt we were complete and ended the session by thanking our guides and closing sacred space.

Chapter 12

Past Lives

THE RESEARCH LITERATURE ON PAST lives is clear and compelling, indicating that reincarnation is a real phenomenon. This is bolstered by the fact that reincarnation is accepted knowledge in many cultures worldwide, the major exception being our modern Western one. Moreover, researchers are accumulating evidence that our other lifetimes can actually influence the incarnation that one currently inhabits. Dr. Stanislav Grof states in his book *When the Impossible Happens: Adventures in Non-Ordinary Realities,* "The existence of past-life experiences with all their remarkable characteristics is an unquestionable fact that can be verified by any serious researcher who is sufficiently open-minded and interested to check the evidence. It is also clear that there is no plausible explanation for these phenomena within the conceptual framework of mainstream psychiatry and psychology."[11]

I think Dr. Grof's statement explains why mainstream science continues to reject the accumulated data on past lives. There is no <u>materialistic</u> explanation for this spiritual event, which is outside of our three-dimensional reality. Add to that simple disbelief that such a process could occur and hubris that if it were true, science would have already shown it to exist. Since no one has yet explained how reincarnation might work, it has been categorically denied.

Our unwavering focus on linear time represents another problem. Accounts from many people who have had near-death experiences indicate that there really are no "past" lives—that all of our countless lives are happening at the same "time" in the eternal now. In other words, there is no past nor future in the higher realms. I agree with this understanding, since it concurs with the teachings of mysticism which state that time as we know it only exists in our physical dimension; the higher dimensions exist in an Eternal Now. All lives existing in an Eternal Now readily explains how clients can visit and work with numerous lifetimes within a single session of the shamanic journey.

It is difficult for us to wrap our minds around this concept, immersed as we are in compellingly linear biological and geological time. It is much easier to think of other lifetimes as past lives rather than simultaneous ones—therefore, I refer to these other lives as *past lives*. Notably, all spirit guides clearly understand what is meant by the term *past life*, and they immediately take clients into the one that is affecting their current life. I have never had a client report experiencing a future life or describe living in fantastic and futuristic scenes, and I find this to be a very thought-provoking aspect of the Great Mystery. Many people take imaginal journeys into the future to see aspects or features of their lives, yet my understanding is that these are all potential timelines that are not "set" in any manner.

The past-life experiences that clients have in their guided journeys, as I have mentioned, are always generated and facilitated by spirit guides. They are continually a surprise to me, yet many of my clients have had experiences, or at least inklings of the past lives they are guided into in their journeys. From my many profound client sessions over the years, as well as my own visits to past lives, I am convinced that past lives, however they work, are real and can be accessed for healing.

Visits to past lives unfold in the guided shamanic journey whether or not the client believes in reincarnation. If that is where the presenting issue originated, the guide will take them there. I avoid making leading suggestions to my clients other than in the broadest terms since I have no idea where they might be heading. The destination to which a higher guide transports the journeyer is always a wonder. I trust and rely on these spirit beings to direct and facilitate the content of the healing journey. The helping spirits have always proven to be knowledgeable and forthcoming concerning questions we have asked them, and they are steadfastly focused on serving each person in the highest manner.

By asking the journeyer to report what they are experiencing as it happens in the session, I can follow the events and participate in the interaction with the guide. My role is to keep the journey focused on the client's issues, ensure the journeyer's safety and ask good questions. I sense when the client has entered a past life and direct them to confirm this with the spirit guide. The guide's confirmation and the direct experience of the past life convince the participant it is real. Although rationally inexplicable, the healing that accrues to the client through past-life repair work is immense, and fosters resolution and restoration that would be difficult to achieve in any other way. The overwhelmingly positive results and feedback I have received from clients reinforce the value of using this potent approach to energy healing.

* * *

Eva was a delightful 11-year-old with an inquisitive nature and a marked ability to perceive energy and the spirit realm. In working with her previously, I found that she could follow the steps and engage with the shamanic journey. Eva's mother had called to tell me that Eva wanted to meet her power animal and asked if I could facilitate this for her. I told her we could almost certainly accomplish a meeting with one of her animal allies.

It had been a while since I had seen Eva. She was taller and dressed in a rose-colored sweatshirt and pants. I welcomed her into my healing room, where she immediately noticed that my altar had changed; it now contained many more feather and crystal tools. We stood beside it to open sacred space and then called in our spiritual support. I did the series of initial cleansings and detected very little debris in her aura. Eva assured me that she was cleansing herself regularly, using the tools I had given her at her last visit. We then prepared for the guided journey, and she was soon comfortably stretched out on a pad next to the altar. I put a small jade jaguar in her left hand as an animal ally to accompany her on the journey and closed the room's curtains.

I began the visualization process and then led her down the steps into the unconscious. Once she was through the gateway, I guided her to call in her power animal. Nothing seemed to be happening at first; then suddenly, she exclaimed there was a butterfly in front of her. I asked if it had a color, and she replied that it did not, but quickly added, "Yes, it's pink." We ascertained that Butterfly was of the light and was her power animal for the journey. In my experience, it is unusual to have an insect as a power animal, but it was in this case, and Butterfly proved to be an expert guide.

I wanted to give Eva an idea of the kinds of things a power animal can do, so I suggested she ask Butterfly to take her to a past life that she could explore. There was a pause, and Eva reported that everything was dark. She gradually became aware of seeing some black and white forms in the distance. I encouraged her to ask Butterfly to augment her perception, and she told me that now she could see they were buildings. I urged her to continue walking forward, and the scene opened up to show her a grassy park surrounded by many multistory brick row houses. She described seeing a number of children playing in the park but added that she recognized herself sitting alone on a bench watching the other children play.

After a pause, Eva commented that she was a nine-year-old boy in that lifetime, and then the story of that life began to unfold in her awareness. The boy's family had been forced to move from their lovely house in the countryside to a new place in this crowded, dingy city. The boy had a sister and a father, but his mother had died a short while ago. Eva could feel some sadness in the boy, but the emotion was not very strong—in fact, the boy was not feeling much of anything.

Eva was transported into the house where the boy lived and described going through it, looking at the myriad objects inside. She realized the boy was not only sad but was also acting out because of his pain and confusion over his mother's death. We asked Butterfly if there was something for Eva to learn from this lifetime, and Butterfly replied that "the lesson is to accept things as they are in life." I suggested Eva ask Butterfly if there was anything she could give her past self to help his situation. Butterfly instructed her to tell the boy what she had just been told, which she did. We asked Butterfly if there was anything else we needed to do in this past life, and she answered, "No, you are here to observe."

I directed Eva to ask Butterfly to take her to another past life where there was an issue affecting her in her current life. There was a pause while the new scene unfolded, and Eva abruptly reported seeing a battlefield amid a fierce battle. She saw a man, a soldier on that field, and he was feeling deep despair. "He is hiding behind a big rock because he is over-whelmed," she reported. The soldier had just witnessed the killing of his best buddy and had suddenly thrown down his gun and refused to fight anymore. She could feel that he was filled with unbearable grief and was frozen in his horror of it all.

I asked Eva if she wanted to help her former self in this past life, to which she replied she most definitely did. I directed her to ask Butterfly to please clear whatever was blocking the man from feeling his intense grief and his vital energy in that critical moment. Butterfly replied that it could be done and immediately proceeded to clear it. We both felt a great surge of energy moving through us, and Eva experienced immense grief welling up inside her. She confided that she wasn't sure if she was making this whole story up or not because the feelings were almost unbearable. I counseled her to keep going with these feelings. Then she started crying as the dam broke, and all the emotional energy began flowing again in both her present and past lives. We paused for a while to let these energies run their course, and I encouraged her to express all her emotions freely.

A few minutes later, Eva reported that she was unexpectedly back again with the nine-year-old boy. She realized that he had blocked all of his emotions to protect himself from the trauma of his mother's death. He had continued to suppress his feelings for his entire life, even on the battlefield where he witnessed his best friend dying. She said it was now clear that she was witnessing the same past life at two different life stages, child and adult.

Eva announced that since the painful feelings had just been set free in her soldier self, she now knew how to help the nine-year-old self release his emotions, too. She took the initiative to help him, revealing that she had just given him a big hug, which had caused his block to dissolve. He began to cry, and along with his tears, all his pent-up emotions flowed once again. Eva stayed with him until the intensity subsided and he became calm once more. When I asked her how she was feeling, she replied that she was delighted to help herself in this past life. She thought it was vitally important to help her past self in healing his suffering. I agreed it was important work and assured her that it would change her present life, too.

Next, I directed Eva to ask if there were any fragments of herself that we could retrieve at this time, to which Butterfly answered, "No." We then asked if there was anything else we needed to do, and Butterfly replied that the journey was complete. Eva then asked Butterfly to take her back to the gateway, which she instantly did. At this point, Butterfly revealed her name to Eva, confirmed that she was her power animal, and vowed to always be with her. Eva told me she was happy and excited to have met her power animal and was looking forward to meeting her again in future journeys.

When Eva was ready to return, I guided her back into this reality and waited until she was sitting up and fully present in the room. She handed the jaguar effigy back to me and said it had been comforting to have him with her. Her tears were long gone, and she was in a calm and happy mood from successfully helping her past self. I encouraged her to reflect on what she had witnessed in her journey, and to think about how it related to her in this lifetime.

To commemorate Eva's new power animal and past-life experience, I gave her a small bronze-colored stone carved in the shape of a butterfly. She loved her new talisman and caressed it before putting it in her pocket. I felt she was ready to undertake shamanic journeys on her own and gave her simple instructions to follow so she could again work with her remarkable ally. Eva said she was eager to journey more with Butterfly and thanked me for introducing her to her power animal. I commended her on the healing work she had done and filled her aura with blessings and prayers. We then thanked our spiritual support and closed sacred space.

* * *

There are numerous books by credible researchers documenting many thousands of case studies of people being taken back through past lives and past deaths using hypnotherapy. Much research has explored not only past lives but also what happens in the spirit realms between incarnations. These case studies, of what is called the "life between lives state," contain a wealth of information that matches ancient spiritual wisdom. Furthermore, the accounts of thousands of hypnotized subjects from different backgrounds and cultures reinforce and concur with this information. Modern science should no longer ignore these extensive data and insights into life after physical death. Expanding evidence-based therapeutic modalities to include past-life therapy could accomplish significant healing for many, particularly in those individuals facing impending death.

The accounts of people who have experienced either extended or multiple near-death experiences are also worthy of serious scientific study. These incidents contribute to our knowledge and understanding of the nature of consciousness, our multiple lives and the soul's purpose for incarnating. It is time for conventional medical and psychological practice to embrace both near-death data and quantum discoveries. We need to tap into the expanded field of consciousness rather than consider thoughts, awareness, and even consciousness itself to be limited to and generated by the human brain.

* * *

Charles, a new referral, called one day to ask me a series of healing-related questions. He said his friend Fred, who had worked with me a few years previously, had given him my name as someone who could access spiritual information. We chatted on the phone for a while, and I asked him what issues he wanted to address. He replied that he had an enlarged prostate and thought maybe a spiritual approach might heal this condition. He confided that he was bothered by the symptoms and wanted to diminish them. I told him we very likely could get some clarity on this from his spirit guides.

Charles appeared right on time for his session. He was a tall, pleasant, middle-aged man dressed simply in a white shirt and jeans. I ushered him to my healing room and gave him a general overview of the work we would do. He was happy to participate in the ceremony of opening sacred space and calling upon our spiritual support and told me that he felt the energy shift in the room. I explained that I would begin with simple energy cleansings, and carried out a series of them on his aura as he stood beside the altar. He had several layers of thick, sticky energies, which I removed and discharged into the ground.

The next step was to undertake the energy extraction process, so I sat him in front of the altar on a large cushion. While using my tourmaline extraction stone, Charles reported that he could feel considerable inky energy leaving his body and entering the stone. I guided him to discharge that energy into my altar and clear the stone with spicy floral waters. I explained that he could do these extractions on his own by finding the proper stone and following the process, which I again outlined for him.

I then gave Charles a summary of the shamanic journey and told him he would be talking to me throughout the process. He opted to lie down for it, and after making sure he was comfortable and relaxed, I darkened the room. Then I led him slowly down the steps into the unconscious and through the gateway. When I directed him to call in a higher guide, one immediately appeared, and we determined that this being was of the light and the appropriate helping spirit for the journey.

Next, I directed Charles to ask his guide to take him to the root cause of his prostate problems. Charles was surprised that the spirit being appeared to be very well informed about this condition. He advised Charles to pay more attention to his "spicy food intake, especially to hot peppers, black pepper, wasabi, horseradish and ginger, all of which are inflammatory." I suggested that Charles ask if it would be of benefit for him to see an Ayurvedic practitioner. The spirit guide replied that the acupuncturist Charles was seeing was already on top of this condition and would be his best resource.

Probing further, I asked Charles if he was aware of the information his spirit helper was telling him about spicy foods. He admitted that he knew some of it but had not changed his habits because he didn't think it was significant. I encouraged him to listen closely to this knowledgeable being and seriously consider what he was saying. I then recommended that Charles ask if there were any emotional, mental or physical causes related to his prostate condition, and the guide replied that all three were involved.

Upon hearing this, I suggested that Charles ask to see more details of the emotional factors first. The higher being informed him that he had a long-standing habit of restricting and suppressing his emotions, particularly with family members. After a pause, Charles revealed that the spirit helper had given him specific and detailed instructions on how to let his emotions come and go, as well as how to release difficult ones. This discussion focused mainly on his feelings about his sister. I asked if he was aware of the information his guide was disclosing. He said he knew his relationship with his sister was a significant problem, and he had many emotional issues with her to resolve. I encouraged him to make this a priority and, further, to give voice to his commitment to do it. He responded by stating aloud that he would make working with his emotions a priority in his life.

Moving on to address the mental aspects of his condition, Charles asked for an overview of them. The higher guide showed him his persistent habit of obsessive sexual attraction toward women, especially his fixation on the sexual contacts he had had in his younger days. I asked if he was aware of this habit, and he admitted he was. He knew the trait was engrained but thought it had nothing to do with his health. His spirit helper assured him it did and told Charles he could help him with this unhealthy preoccupation if he would be willing to work on it. Charles replied that he was and welcomed any assistance this being could give him. I asked him if he could easily communicate with his guide on an ongoing basis, and he felt confident that he could and would.

Next, I suggested Charles ask for more insight into the physical causes of his condition. His spirit guide replied that these occurred in both his current incarnation and past lives, and he needed to address them all. The cause, his higher being explained, was that Charles had indulged too much in sex. I encouraged Charles to ask to visit the past lives to clear the archived energies from those first, which he then did.

After a few moments, Charles reported that he was viewing a past life where he had been the owner of a brothel and could see the entire pattern of that lifetime laid out before him. He understood that he had badly abused his body during that life. The guide informed him that there were numerous similar past lives, which formed a persistent pattern of behavior that had continued into the present.

I prompted Charles to ask if his helping spirit could clear the accumulated energy of these past lives and his deep-rooted pattern of overindulgence all at once, rather than clear each lifetime one by one. The guide confirmed that he could and immediately began to fulfill this request. In a surprised tone, Charles announced he could physically feel the clearing of these past-life energetic deposits—it was as if a very heavy weight had been lifted from him. Within moments, his higher guide reported that the entire past-life clearing was complete and that he had replaced the oppressive energy deposits with balanced, healthy vitality. Charles said he was now feeling considerably lighter and was deeply impressed by the realization that he had been carrying lifetimes of such dense, burdensome energies.

We then asked for information on clearing the unhealthy physical consequences of this current life. The guide advised Charles that the best way was for him to perform a small ritual, and instructed him to write down on a single sheet of paper the names of all the women with whom he had been sexually involved. Once completed, he was to "burn the list of names in a ceremony honoring everyone involved." I asked Charles if this made sense to him and whether he had any questions about what he needed to do. "No," he replied. "It's all very clear." The spirit being then had Charles pledge aloud that he would perform the ritual. I agreed that it was a wise assignment and would be powerfully healing for everyone.

Next, I encouraged Charles to ask if his spirit helper would be readily available to him for any continuing work. The higher being replied that he was always available whenever Charles called upon him. I then questioned Charles about his willingness to request spiritual help whenever any of these or other issues arose in his everyday life, and he unhesitatingly affirmed that he would.

After a few moments of silence, Charles reported that the guide had just admonished him "to lighten up, to laugh more, to allow, and not take life so seriously." The being further explained that Charles could significantly reduce the prostate constriction by introducing more humor into his life. Again, the guide stressed that cutting down on spicy foods would reduce the heat in his body, which would reduce the inflammation and swelling he was experiencing. Charles repeated that he now understood the problem and promised to change his diet immediately. I confirmed that this was pivotal and assured him it would make a difference in his health.

The higher guide reaffirmed that he was always available but said that Charles had the habit of resisting turning to him for help. I underscored the importance and good fortune of having such a knowledgeable, helpful guide who was so easily accessible. Charles promised to change his habit, ask his guide for help regularly and continue to build their relationship.

I then suggested Charles might inquire whether any of the stressful energy he carried was a result of cultural programming. The spirit being replied that it was entirely Charles' personal material and that he alone was responsible for it, to which Charles wholeheartedly agreed.

At that point, the helper spirit informed us that we had covered all we could for the session. I directed Charles to ask to return to the gateway, and instantly he was there. I reminded him to thank his guide and remember his promise to call on him regularly for recommendations and advice. Charles reiterated his intention to do it. When he was ready to return, I brought him back up the steps into the present moment. After a few minutes, he sat up and I opened the curtains to let in more light.

We then had a lengthy discussion about spirit guides. Charles had long been aware of having a guide and could easily communicate with him, but had not truly realized what a blessing this represented until today. He said he felt differently now because he understood how this relationship could work and benefit him. Charles was genuinely pleased with everything he had learned in his session. He saw his life in a new light and was determined to carry out his assignments. I congratulated him for making good progress and encouraged him to continue healing himself by changing his old habits.

Charles looked considerably more relaxed and comfortable in his body than he had before the journey, and I mentioned that he looked much lighter. He said he also felt younger and more alive now. I reminded him about his ceremonial assignment and underlined that a well-orchestrated ceremony had considerable healing power and would produce tangible physical results. Charles thanked me for facilitating his session and reiterated that he already felt a great sense of relief from everything he had experienced in his journey. We then thanked our spiritual support team and closed sacred space.

Chapter 13

Speaking with the Deceased

SINCE TIME IMMEMORIAL, AND WITHIN myriad civilizations, humans have communicated with deceased family and friends, among many others. Nearly all world religions promote belief in an afterlife with teachings on what happens after death. They assure the living that those who have gone before are still connected to us and are aware of all that happens on Earth. For example, the modern cultures of Japan, Korea and parts of Africa continue to practice ancient ancestor rituals based on the understanding that the dead will greatly benefit from the actions of their living descendants. The living, in turn, are blessed and protected by the ancestors who have been honored. There is no barrier between the living and the dead in these ancient traditions. They experience their ancestors as freely communicating and interacting with living family members.

Many Indigenous cultures highly esteem those who can communicate with the departed. A quick review of the popularity of mediums who can speak with the dead shows us that many people in the U.S. currently value this ability, too. Studies have shown that from 25 to 40 percent of people in the United States believe they have had an encounter with a deceased person. "An encounter" was defined as physical—tactile, auditory or olfactory—in nature. If we broaden this definition to include visual sightings, dreams and intuitive encounters, the percentage would undoubtedly be considerably higher. Communication with the deceased usually involves contact with departed humans, but many accounts exist of people communicating with their dead pets. Most importantly, people who have had contact experiences overwhelmingly report that their encounter with the deceased resulted in positive impacts on their mental and emotional well-being.

Modern researchers are discovering that the act of communicating with friends or relatives who have passed can help resolve the grief, regrets and confusion of those left behind. Communication with the dead can also convey a sense of peace, allowing the individual to move on with their life in a meaningful way. Many people regularly speak to the departed at cemeteries, offering prayers and flowers and letting the deceased know what has been happening to loved ones since their passing. Surveys have shown the practice of talking to photos of deceased family members is extremely common.

Many people who have lost a loved one say that they still have a palpable sense of love and connection with that person. It is also common for individuals to reveal that they feel they are being watched over, protected, blessed, forgiven and guided by a deceased relative or friend. Having the ability or opportunity to speak to the departed can provide deep healing on emotional and psychological levels. This is especially true for those who were not able to communicate with the person before they passed. The following case study illustrates the healing that can come from the simple act of having an opportunity to connect with the deceased.

* * *

My long-time friend Teresa called to ask if I had time to see her co-worker, Marta. She was calling from their workplace and said this was something of an emergency. Teresa explained that Marta was so distraught by the recent news of her father's passing that she could not concentrate or do her work. I cleared my schedule and told Marta to come as soon as possible.

Half an hour later, Marta arrived. She was a petite young woman with black hair and deep brown eyes. I ushered her into my healing room, making sure she was comfortably seated at my altar. As I spoke with her, she explained that she had learned of her father's death the previous day and, although she had tried, she had not been able to talk to him before he died. "And now it is too late," she added tearfully. I asked her to tell me more about herself and her relationship with her father. She replied that her father had left her mother when she was a very young girl and had returned to Mexico, where he had been living with his current wife ever since.

Marta admitted that she and her father had had little contact over the years, but when she heard he was dying, she knew she had to talk to him. She had telephoned him, wanting to say her final goodbye. However, his wife would not let her speak to him, even though he was in an adjacent room. The following day he passed away, and when Marta heard the news, she was overcome with grief and regret that she had lost the opportunity to talk to him. She was so upset that she was unable to concentrate on her job or even think about anything else. She was in tears as she said this, reinforcing my desire to help her to speak with her father.

I encouraged Marta to tell me, in greater detail, about her relationship with her father. She recounted many things from her childhood, but what bothered her most was that she had been very angry at him for abandoning her and her mother. She explained that her mother eventually found a boyfriend with whom the mother became involved, resulting in his moving in with them. Unfortunately, this man was an exploitative person and sexually abused Marta for years when she was a young girl. For many years, she harbored great resentment toward her father for not protecting her from this predator and blamed him for everything that had happened.

I listened carefully to Marta and then outlined how we would proceed with the session. She stated that she was ready and willing to participate. First, I performed the series of energy cleansings of her aura, sweeping several layers of heavy, blocking energy into my altar. When I asked if she could perceive these energies, she said she did not feel them directly but later commented that she felt like a door somewhere inside had opened a little and more light came in.

We then moved on to address the entities I was sure Marta carried. I explained what I meant by this term, and she acknowledged that they exist. As I guided her, she discovered and expelled half a dozen entities that she had sheltered for many years. Even though several of these were very ominous beings, Marta had no difficulty removing them and having the guides take them away. We both had the sense that these entities had come into her during her childhood abuse, and once they were gone, she reported feeling calmer and more hopeful.

Next, I gave Marta an overview of the shamanic journey, including telling her we would call in the spirit of her father. She lay down on a pad beside the altar with an eye pillow and a blanket. I led her into a deeply relaxed state and then down the steps into the unconscious. When I directed her to call in her higher guide, a large, luminous being appeared to her. After determining that he was truly of the light and appropriate for the session, I told her to ask him to bring in her father in his etheric body. Moments later, Marta's surprised response was, "Oh, he's here," as he came fully into her presence.

I explained to Marta that this was her opportunity to tell him everything she had wanted to say before he passed. She spoke to him with great emotion and many tears for several minutes and then reported that her father was happy and smiling. He was glad to see her and to hear everything she was telling him. She felt tremendous surprise and relief at actually being in the presence of her deceased father and able to converse with him directly. "This has been a huge blessing for both my father and me," she exclaimed and then dove back into their conversation.

After a while, the discussion subsided, and I gently encouraged Marta to tell her father how she felt about his deserting her and her mother when she was a child. She was hesitant to bring up this uncomfortable topic and risk ruining the festive mood. I reminded her that this was her best moment to heal her long-held resentment and anger. I urged her to use this precious time with him to let him know all that had happened to her because he left.

Marta paused for a few minutes to consider her feelings. She then told him about all the abuse she had endured by not having a father there to protect her and how much she had suffered. Marta confessed feeling anger toward him for many years and said she still carried some bitterness about it. When she finished speaking, I asked her how her father was doing with this disclosure. She replied, "He is not smiling anymore. He is very sad."

I recommended that Marta allow her father to experience his distress about the pain his actions had caused her. She began to cry again as he assured her that he had not known about any of this. He was truly sorry to hear what had happened and apologized sincerely to her. It had never been his intention to hurt her in any way, he said. It was the marriage that didn't work, he explained, and it was not her fault. He then told her he loved her dearly and asked her to please forgive him.

Upon hearing this, Marta hesitated for a few minutes, unsure of what to do. I let her sit in silence with all her feelings until she was ready to decide. Shortly, Marta announced that she could forgive him. She had told him all she needed to say and heard his sincere responses. She assured her father that she honestly forgave him and was ready to move on with her life without any more anger at him.

Their conversation continued for a while longer as Marta gave her father news of other events and people in her life. At last, she indicated they had finished talking "for the time being." I pointed out that, with the help of her higher guide, she and her father could reconnect again any time she wanted to speak to him. Her luminous guide quickly confirmed this and said he would always be available to her for any help and guidance she needed.

I directed Marta to say goodbye to her father and ask the spirit being to return him to wherever he belonged. She stated that he had disappeared into a bright light, and then she sighed deeply. She felt greatly relieved to have spoken with him; it was as if an enormous burden had been lifted off of her and replaced by feelings of peace and tranquility. I told her I was glad to hear it and pleased that her disclosure to her father had gone so well.

Next, I suggested that Marta ask if there were any soul fragments that we could retrieve during the journey. The spirit guide advised us that many shards had split off during her sexual abuse, and they were ready to be reunited. They appeared as numerous small lights, like little stars in the darkness. I encouraged her to request that they be returned to her as a group, and, as she made this appeal, the luminous being helped her gather them up as a cluster and reincorporate them into her body.

I gave Marta a detailed explanation of what these fragments represented and made specific suggestions about caring for them. I told her she might have more soul pieces that she could collect in the future with the guide's assistance. The light being again assured her he would always be available to her whenever she called upon him, and she expressed her gratitude to him.

We paused for a while to let Marta integrate her experience of the soul retrieval. The spirit helper then advised us that we had done enough work for the day. I asked Marta to request that he take her back to the gateway, and she instantly found herself there. She thanked her luminous guide once more for all his help, promising to call upon him in the future. I asked if she was ready to return and then brought her back up the steps into my healing space.

I was stunned to see the transformation in Marta and hardly recognized her. The tears, grief and disabling sadness were gone, and before me was a radiant, happy and serene young woman. Her eyes were shining, and she positively beamed with joy. I, too, was joyous for Marta and profoundly moved to have witnessed the incredible healing power of this session. Having the opportunity to finally tell her father everything she needed to say to him and to hear his genuine response, she said, "was like a miracle." I told her I felt the same way and commended her for having the courage to speak her truth in a difficult situation. She admitted that, even though it had been hard, she was extremely glad that she had been honest with him and had released her heavy burden.

Using high vibration floral waters, feathers and prayers, I filled her aura with an uplifting and sustaining vibrancy to support her integration. To commemorate her journey and her courage, I gave her a talisman from my altar. We chatted for a while, and she told me more details of the conversation with her father. She then thanked me profusely for giving her the incredible opportunity to speak with him, and I replied that it was my privilege to help her. We then thanked all the guides, closed our sacred space, and she left to return to work.

A few days later, I heard from Teresa that no one at her workplace could believe that Marta was the same person who had left distraught and in tears earlier in the day. She excitedly told me that everyone had remarked on the miraculous change in Marta's appearance and behavior. I confided that I was as astonished as anyone to witness the magical transformation that had occurred and was delighted to hear the confirmation from her co-workers. I added that I was deeply grateful I had chosen to pursue energy healing work and thanked Teresa for referring Marta to me.

* * *

Contact and communication with deceased ancestors have great potential to heal many unaddressed issues that continue to affect both the living and the dead. Those who have incarnated before us can be a source of great wisdom to the living, allowing us to learn from the experiences, mistakes and perspectives they have amassed.

Key words in any practice of communing with the deceased are *family, relatives, friends* and *ancestors*. It is crucial to distinguish the long-accepted and mutually beneficial practice of communicating with one's ancestors from that which is called *Spiritism*. Spiritism, along with séances, was very popular in the 1800s and is still practiced by many in the present. The term refers to the practice of engaging in intentional open communication with the dead (seen as being in the spirit realm), regardless of who they are, and usually without any safety parameters. The act of randomly opening oneself to unknown and potentially unhealthy deceased beings is not wise. Aside from departed humans, numerous other spirit beings are attracted to such activities—many of whom can be troublesome, at best. As I have mentioned, a disincarnate state does not ensure that a being will be knowledgeable, kind, helpful, truthful or benevolent.

Disbelief in a spirit realm is a relatively modern phenomenon. Conventional Western medical science, which continues to deny the continuity of consciousness after death and even denigrates and ridicules those who embrace it as fact, is beginning to change. Scientific attitudes labeling communication with the dead as magical thinking, delusion or superstition are being questioned, and it is heartening to see new research encouraging this practice and reporting its benefits. Although charlatans and impostors may abound, there are far too many credible examples documented in modern times to dismiss conversing with the dead as fantasy or fraud. I have not worked with a single person who felt their communication with a deceased person was make-believe or "all in their head." Our societal beliefs are spiraling back to reincorporate past cultural wisdom as our spiritual evolution progresses, and this is inspiring.

* * *

Jane, a middle-aged professional woman, was a client with whom I had worked previously. She called to tell me she had a list of questions to which she wanted answers. I asked what she had in mind, and she replied that the first one was to find out why she had such a strong resistance to doing things that would be good for her. "Like yoga," she said, as an example. Secondly, she wanted to know why she harbored a large amount of barely-suppressed anger and fear. Jane added that she still had issues with her mother-in-law, who had been deceased for many years, and wanted to examine that. Next, she mentioned that she was also aware she had "some brain chemistry issues" from infancy and wanted to heal them. I replied that I felt we could get some clear answers to all these questions, and we scheduled a session for the following week.

I greeted Jane and gave her a welcoming hug. She was dressed all in purple, which was a flattering color for her. Standing and facing my altar, we opened sacred space and called in our spiritual support. I gave her a review of the work we would be doing and began with the series of energy cleansings. After cleansing some dense clogging energies from her aura and determining that she felt lighter, we proceeded to check for entities. We had removed several of them during her previous session, and no new ones appeared, which was good news.

Jane lay down on a pad, put on her blindfold and began to relax as I pulled the shades in the room. I guided her in a slow descent into the unconscious and after she passed through the gateway, she called for a higher guide. Jane is Buddhist and reported that she saw the form of the Buddha come clearly into her vision. I directed her to ask the Buddha if he was to be the guide for today's session; he replied that he was simply there to oversee the work we were doing. I then asked Jane to call in another guide and, as she did this, Mother Mary immediately appeared. We questioned Mother Mary to be sure she was the appropriate guide for the journey, and she confirmed that she was.

I directed Jane to ask Mary to take her to the root of her problems with anger and fear, as well as her brain chemistry issues. Moments later, she saw a scene of herself as an infant sitting all alone in a crib and feeling utterly despondent. Her mother was nowhere in sight, making it clear that Jane was a neglected child. Mary emphasized this neglect and explained that much of it had happened at critical times in Jane's life, leaving a deep imprint on her psyche.

I suggested Jane request healing for the neglect she had suffered as an infant, and she asked Mary to help heal this serious wound. Without delay, Mary reached into the crib, picked up the infant Jane, and then sat down in a chair, lovingly holding the baby in her arms. Jane reported with amazement that immense love, acceptance, and feelings of being cherished were flowing into both her infant and adult selves simultaneously. We paused for many minutes to let the healing energies soak into her.

Mary then assured Jane she is always loved and that there has never been a moment when any person has not been loved and held by Divine Beings. Jane said she was astonished by what Mary told her and what she felt coming from Mary's heart. We both felt unconditionally held in these sublime energies, and I could feel they were deeply repairing Jane's wounds. She asked Mary if these beautiful energies would fully alleviate her anger, and Mary assured her that this anger was healed. Jane then wholeheartedly thanked her guide for the profound and loving restoration.

Following this, I guided Jane to ask Mary to bring in her mother-in-law, who appeared before her in an instant. Jane reported that her mother-in-law appeared to be in a light body, and said she was shining. I suggested that Jane ask to see an expanded scope of what had occurred between them and what needed to be healed. She narrated the story, telling me her mother-in-law had moved in with Jane and her husband many years ago. The mother-in-law did not have much longer to live and wanted to be with her son when she died. Jane explained that she had been eight months pregnant when the mother-in-law arrived, and it had been an extremely stressful time for her.

I encouraged Jane to tell her mother-in-law exactly how she felt about what had transpired during that time. After a few minutes, Jane reported that she had said all she needed to her mother-in-law, and I then urged her to ask her mother-in-law to respond. The mother-in-law replied that she had never expected to be cared for by anyone because she had always felt she "was not worth it." This reply acutely struck Jane since it mirrored her own feelings of unworthiness. Furthermore, this was the main rationale she had always given herself about why her mother had neglected her. Jane suddenly realized that her mother-in-law had endured the same kind of infant trauma as she had and that neither of them had ever healed those painful wounds.

Jane could see that her mother-in-law had never held any grudges or judgment against her, as she had always imagined. She realized that she had made this up by turning her experience of her mother-in-law in on herself, reflecting her childhood feelings of abandonment. Jane confessed to judging herself poorly—for many years—for being resentful of her mother-in-law and not caring for her as she should have. Moments later, she added that it was now obvious that they both had employed the same basic coping patterns throughout their lives, and that these had resulted from having identical early childhood wounds.

I suggested that Jane ask her mother-in-law if she wanted to receive energy healing for the embedded trauma she still carried. The woman's light body glowed and she quickly replied that she would welcome it. Mary immediately cleared the pain and healed the deep-seated injuries, much to the mother-in-law's surprise. We all thanked Mary for this crucial healing and paused to let it integrate. Jane remarked that she felt a large internal energetic shift and realized that Mary had simultaneously healed them both. Mary advised us that this part of Jane's healing journey was now complete and returned the mother-in-law to the realm where she resided.

At that point, I remembered Jane's concerns about her brain chemistry and suggested she ask if Mary could heal the imbalances that had been created during her infancy. Mary immediately put her hands on either side of Jane's head, bringing it close to her lips. She gently blew into Jane's head, and Jane reported that soothing and cleansing energy filled her awareness. She said it gave her a feeling of deep peace and serenity, and Mary whispered, "Your brain is healed."

Mary then counseled Jane to remember a phrase she had received during her recent spiritual retreat: "Cherish yourself just as you are." Jane remembered these words but had not taken them to heart as something to be applied literally. She now saw their purpose and agreed to incorporate this phrase into her daily meditation practice. Mary encouraged her in her decision and asked Jane to call on her if she ever needed help remembering it.

I reminded Jane that she wanted to ask about her resistance to doing yoga and other activities she knew would benefit her. Mary explained that this was due to Jane's holding "terror in the body." I suggested she ask to see the source of this terror, and Mary opened a scene in which Jane saw herself as a lively young teen. She watched an episode unfold in which she had dislocated both of her knees. Witnessing the event again made her realize that ever since that time, she had held a strong belief that she could not depend on her body; as she sadly put it, "My body let me down." She had suffered from her dislocated knees for several years, even using crutches to get around, and eventually had undergone surgery to correct the problem. She admitted that her knees had not given her any trouble since, but she was still carrying her fear and anger from that time.

Jane asked Mary to please clear this stored anguish. Almost immediately, she could feel that it was entirely healed. I had an intuition that there was a past-life energetic charge attached to the knee issue and suggested Jane ask about it. Mary responded by taking Jane back to a past life, where she reported with some alarm that she was witnessing herself being burned at the stake. As she watched herself burning and feeling the terror of this horrific death, she realized that the fear and pain she had experienced in that life was still remarkably present in her psyche in this lifetime. Jane asked if this terror could be cleared or at least decreased, and Mary's unexpected answer was, "No, this is something we all need to accept. Death is part of life; we all die." We both agreed that this was a true—but very puzzling—response, and Jane decided she would sit with this advice in her meditations to see what unfolded.

Mary then helped Jane see how her emotions were connected: experiencing terror led to embodying fear, which then led to anger, and this finally became embedded as resistance. Jane reported that her resistance to doing what was good for her body now made complete sense, and she could see it was simply a bad habit that she could dismantle. She asked if Mary would be available every day to help her as she let go of this habit, and Mary's reply was, "I am always here for you."

After a few moments of silence, Jane surprised me by confiding that she now felt even more anger. I encouraged her to ask to be taken to the source of this anger, and she told me she was now at the scene of her father's death. The entire episode was playing before her like a movie, and she described it as it unfolded. Her father had been in the bathroom when he suffered a major stroke; unconscious, he had fallen against the door, completely blocking it. Only 17 at the time, Jane had been terribly frightened by this shocking event. She knew her father was dying but did not want to go into the bathroom. The only thing she could think of to do was to call 911.

Hearing the noise, her mother came running in from another room. Jane told her what she thought had happened, but neither one tried to get into the bathroom. Jane remembered her immensely conflicting feelings—she felt she should be there with her father as he lay dying, but at the same time, she was angry and resentful of his behavior over the years. He had been highly abusive and violent with the whole family, especially her mother. She admitted that she always felt the need to protect herself from him.

As Jane relived this scene, she perceived that she and her mother were having identical conflicting emotions. Both of them felt extremely guilty for not being with him, but they were also intensely angry that he was such a monster. Jane admitted that she wanted him to die to get him out of her life. At this point, she realized that her only mode of coping with the raging, conflicted feelings had been to turn them in on herself, and this had become her lifelong pattern.

Mary explained to Jane that she is exceptionally empathic. She had been feeling her own emotions in addition to those of her mother and father. Jane considered this, recognizing that she had been emotionally enmeshed with her entire family all her life and had never had any boundaries. I asked her if she knew what boundaries were, and she replied that, even though she was seeing that she lacked them, she was not sure what they actually were.

We spent several minutes discussing boundaries—how to perceive them and how Jane could set healthy ones for herself. She agreed to start by being solely responsible for herself and her feelings—and not for anyone else's. She admitted that this was hard and confusing and acknowledged that it might take her a while, but she was committed to accomplishing it. We asked Mary to please help heal any aspect of the boundary issue that involved Jane's brain chemistry and make it easier for her to make the necessary changes. Mary again took Jane's head in her hands and gently blew her healing energies into it. Jane immediately thanked her, telling both of us it felt wonderfully restoring.

At that point, Jane began reflecting on what she had experienced in the journey. She realized that much of her resentment toward her mother-in-law was, in truth, connected to unresolved emotions about her father. Overall, she said she felt much better about her life and herself but could see she had other issues to address that were now arising. Mary informed her that additional work would have to wait for a future session because we had done enough for one day. She promised Jane she would always be present and help her with all her concerns, and Jane expressed her deep gratitude for Mary's love, care and guidance.

I then directed Jane to request to be taken back to the gateway, and she was immediately there. She thanked Mary once more for all the healing she had facilitated and told her she was excited about the work they would be doing together in the future. When she was ready, I brought her back up the steps into our ordinary reality.

Jane and I talked for quite a while as she continued her integration and grounding. She had a new calmness and ease about her and was smiling a lot as she spoke. She was deeply grateful for the opportunity to get answers to her many questions and for the profound insights and healing she had received. I encouraged her to continue working on her own with Mary's guidance because she had a developed ability to communicate with her guide. Jane replied that she definitely would do that. To end our session, we closed sacred space and thanked all our guides for their service.

* * *

I want to comment on the topic of past-life memories of being burned at the stake. Over the past 40+ years, I have met many people who have memories of dying this way, some in more than one incarnation. It is a frequent past-life theme that emerges in all types of journeys and appears to be especially common in those who have chosen to follow healing professions or are psychically gifted in their present incarnations. Many of them state that the memories they carry "from the burning times" are unusually pervasive in their current lives.

Enormous numbers of people (mostly women) suffered this fate between 600 and 1727 CE. Estimates are that anywhere between tens of thousands and nine million human beings were tortured and killed by burning during this 1100-year span. I suspect the number is closer to the higher end of the range than to the lower one. Given the number of people murdered in this way, it is hardly surprising that many people alive today would have an archived account of such a horrific and brutal end to a past life.

Extremely traumatic deaths can leave a charge or deposit so potent that the effects may endure through many lifetimes. Deaths that are peaceful and do not involve trauma or chaos do not leave unfinished business behind. I feel it is essential we seriously consider, or at least respect, every person's account of a past life since there have been no data presented to counter or invalidate these numerous experiences. The time for ridicule and ignorance regarding the validity of past-life memories is long past.

Chapter 14

Incarnational Planning and Guidance

I HAVE TAKEN NUMEROUS CLIENTS into the state of being that we exist in before we embark on each incarnation. As mentioned previously, this realm is commonly referred to as the life between lives state or LBL. Many informative books have been written detailing thousands of accounts of people being guided through their deaths in a past life and their movement into the "afterlife state," and then following them through the entire LBL episode. Within this LBL state we apparently have myriad experiences, one of which is the planning of our next incarnation. I recommend the books of Michael Newton, PhD, as a good place to begin for those who would like to understand the LBL realm in more depth.

Research into LBLs reveals that each person, along with a team of spiritual advisors, plans their incarnation to include all the main lessons they want to learn, the experiences they would like to have, the karma they want to clear, and any rebalancing or harmonizing of energies that have resulted from past lives or have been inherited. It is my understanding that we are all shown a few different options of bodies and lives that are available to us and allowed to choose which one we prefer. No one is "forced" to incarnate, yet considerable pressure can apparently be put on those who are reluctant to return to Earth School for more training.

Most of the methodologies for the LBL work involve deep, advanced hypnotherapy techniques, provided by seasoned hypnotherapists. This is not necessary for the modality I outline here. What I explore in this chapter is a much simpler process that is oriented toward obtaining information, insight, guidance and options for one's current incarnation through consulting with the guide who helped the client plan it.

I have found that the key is enlisting the appropriate incarnational guide for the journey. There are echelons of spirit beings with different capacities, responsibilities and access to information. What is required for this modality is to employ a higher being who can transport the client into the precise state needed for entering the LBL, or pre-incarnational state. If the person needs to achieve a deeper trance to enter the LBL state, the guide might facilitate that spontaneously. Alternatively, you can direct the client to request the proper trance level if they are having difficulty accessing that stratum of awareness.

The beauty and utility of visiting the LBL state is that it enables us to consult with a masterful being who will be able to assist the client in reviewing their life plan. The guide can inform the person of options, deeper healing and solutions to problems, and even to help renegotiate the contents of what has been called the "soul script." The incarnation guide can also help the client integrate this material and gently bring them back into the regular journey space. This process is a simple and direct method to address questions that cannot be easily answered in other ways, allowing the client to gain valuable insight into life experiences that are generally beyond our reach as incarnated beings.

In some cases, the information presented in the journey to the LBL state does not greatly differ from the "regular" guided shamanic journey. It may be that higher guides who have expanded access to a person's soul states, as well as the capacity to perform the functions requested, are the ones who appear. Or, perhaps, many spirit beings have these abilities but have not been asked to provide this specific viewpoint. However one accesses this information, it generally has a substantial impact on the client.

An example of the depth of information and insight that can be received is highlighted in this next case study.

* * *

June was an elderly woman who was in fragile health due to having leukemia. She had been referred to me by a past client, and I greeted her at the door with a hug. She was petite and very slender, with beautiful silver hair but also an air of exhaustion about her from the severe illness she was facing.

I led her to a seat next to my altar where we chatted a bit about her state of health, her prognosis and how she was feeling about it all. The debilitating effects of chemo and antibiotics were taking a toll, and she described a sensation of deep weakness in her body. She wondered aloud if that meant she would be "dying sooner rather than later." I outlined for her what our session would entail, and she said she was ready.

We then set our sacred space. I performed a few cleansings of her aura before leading her in an extraction with my favorite stone. Then I made sure June was comfortably reclining on cushions with a blanket and eye mask for the journey. Once she was through the gateway, she requested that the Advisor from her life-between-lives state come in. I felt a very large being manifest in the room, but June was unable to sense its presence. I recommended that she ask this luminous guide to augment her capacity to perceive him, and that helped immensely.

Our first request was for June to be taken to her LBL state just before her current incarnation onto earth. This also proved to be a little difficult for June, so we asked the Advisor to please deepen her state of consciousness to allow her to make that transition. June immediately reported feeling like she was sinking into a large pool of warm water.

Suddenly, she exclaimed that she saw blood all over her body, and she felt that her blood had turned against her. This clearly was the leukemia. The diagnosis had terrified her, and she had been having depressive thoughts since her oncologist's callous prediction that she had only six months to live. I directed June to ask her Advisor about the effect of the doctor's decree on her and her outlook on life. The guide stated that the doctor's diagnosis had been delivered with the impact of a curse, and we immediately requested that all adverse results of the pronouncement be cleared.

June admitted having a huge fear of death, which was a major block in trying to move forward. I suggested she ask the Advisor whether it was her own fear, or fear she had inherited from her ancestors. His answer was that June had brought that fear energy from a previous life into this lifetime in order to heal it. "Can I ask for that painful past life to be cleared right now?" June implored. To her relief, the spirit being replied, "Certainly." We then requested a guide who could transform the archive of that life. With a look of surprise, June reported that a fairy godmother with a wand suddenly appeared. She entreated this shining being to transmute the past-life fear of death, and it was instantly cleared.

We asked the Advisor if June's illness was a part of her life plan and his immediate answer was, "Yes!" He explained that its purpose is to test her strength in this lifetime, and acknowledged that it does represent an enormous trial for her. She confessed thinking,"If it gets too hard, I will just leave!" Her higher guide acknowledged that yes, June believes this is an option, but "it is easy to think and hard to do." Apparently, it is not that easy to die.

Our next question was whether June's perception of her illness could be transformed from the current doom and despair into a sense of possibility and openness. The Advisor instantly declared that it was done, and that June would now be able to see and accept the gifts as well as the challenges of her situation.

Earlier, June had explained to me that she was an artist and that this had been her whole life up until becoming depleted by the leukemia. Yet even as she was losing the ability to create her art, she felt driven to continue. "Is this something that is damaging to my health?" she asked. June's parents had been preoccupied with their own lives and had neglected her throughout her childhood. She had become a skilled artist as a way to get her father's attention and approval, and she was quite attached to that persona. The Advisor explained that it was indeed a problem for her because she had developed a false self in order to be loved. Even decades after his death, June's desire to please her father pushed her to keep going in spite of her increasing exhaustion.

When we asked what could be done to resolve the issue, the curt reply was, "Just drop it!" As June began to protest, the spirit guide reiterated that the lesson in this moment is about making a choice. She can choose to let go of her artist identity, or let herself be forced to do it by the debilitating cancer. Faced with this stark reality, June decided to drop all her artwork and see what unfolds.

"What other factors are affecting my healing?" was the next question. Her Advisor pointed out that June tends to take on too much and push herself too hard in most situations. "Your life has to be brought more into balance and harmony," he advised. "You need to learn to let go of some things." He stressed the importance of making deliberate choices rather than letting herself be forced into something she didn't really want.

I asked June what she would most love to do if she could choose anything. She shyly admitted that she dreamed of going to a fancy spa and letting herself be completely pampered. Her Advisor endorsed the idea, saying that it would be a beneficial and restorative adventure for her. He stressed again that June's alternatives are to love and care for herself, or to merely succumb to her illness. "All the healing you do will make whatever time you do have left in this life more valuable and enjoyable," he advised.

June wanted to know if the plan she had made for her current life included the possibility of overcoming her illness. The spirit being confirmed that it did, and went on to provide additional guidance. First of all, it was essential for her to get sufficient rest while undergoing chemotherapy in order to keep her body strong. It was also important to explore new interests that would enhance her mental and emotional well-being. In addition, opportunities for transformation and healing could occur via the many people and situations she would encounter during the course of her treatment. "Looking for all the good things that can come will increase the quality of your life, making it better and better," he advised.

Optimism crept into June's voice. She told me that her husband was learning how to give her the support she needed, and that giving up her art would make it possible to spend more time with her friends. Then she began to think of more options, such as seeing a counselor and joining a support group, and investigating the resources available through the Leukemia Society. Above all, she said, she would choose to speak up and advocate for her needs. "My task is to bring all of this into harmony," she mused, "to be in the flow of life, decrease the speed of my life, and to rest and restore."

The luminous being stated that we had done enough for one day, and assured June that he is available whenever she calls upon him. She reflected that she now felt able to "re-evaluate what I've been doing with more clarity." She asked to be returned to the gateway, and was gently transported there. She thanked her Advisor for his invaluable help, and said good-bye. I guided her up the steps into the light of a newly realized day.

* * *

As with those who have a near-death experience, visiting the LBL state can give us an expanded view of what it means to be human, as well as a deep appreciation for the preciousness of our life in a physical body. In addition to an incarnational overview and awareness of our life plan, it can also present us with a deeper understanding of the connection of our body to our soul. There is even the potential to recognize and connect with others in our soul group who have incarnated with us in this lifetime. Past lives and ancestral healing are other areas that can be highlighted in a review of the soul's plan, along with any other inherited issues. One might also see and understand how karma plays out, not as judgment or punishment, but as a balancing and harmonizing force. I imagine there are many more benefits to this aspect of shamanic journeys that await discovery.

* * *

Karen, a young body worker and spiritual guide, had been referred to me because she felt blocked by something that involved both her ancestors and her past lives. Since her understanding of these issues was murky, I suggested an LBL type of journey. Karen lives outside of the United States, so we opted for a remote session by phone. We began with the usual cleansings, extraction and removal of entities. I then guided her in the journey induction, leading her down the steps and through the gateway.

When Karen called for her incarnational guide, the being who appeared was named Vasan. We confirmed that Vasan was of the light and that she was the appropriate guide to take Karen to the LBL state. We asked the luminous being to put Karen into the proper frequency to travel to the before-life realm. Once there, Karen asked to see an overview of her life plan, which focused on further developing her skills as a healer. This included the healing of specific inherited beliefs and patterns that Karen had chosen to clear. There were also some blocks to her creativity that she wanted to explore.

The main block was in Karen's childhood. Her father had passed away suddenly when Karen was young. As a result, her mother set aside all of her own creative endeavors in order to go to work and support the family. Karen felt that she should also take on more responsibility for her family. She abruptly shuttered her creative abilities, imagination and inspiration, feeling that she could no longer "just be a kid." When we asked how to heal this obstacle, Vasan replied that Karen could revisit her childhood decision to reject her creativity and ask for it to be transformed instead into an openness to whatever creative expression wishes to come through her. Karen happily requested this to be done.

We then moved on to another issue, which concerned ancestral karma in her father's lineage. Vasan revealed that Karen's grandparents had created a pyramid scheme, which resulted in many people being harmed and losing a great deal of money. The consequences of this event were karmic energies of deep shame and guilt, which Karen had chosen to heal during this lifetime. We asked for the best option to clear and resolve this block. Vasan indicated that Karen needs to create a "pyramid of love." Its purpose was to attract and create sufficient "good" to balance the "negative" karma, using the power of love to heal the misuse of power that had occurred.

As this unfolded, Karen glimpsed a memory of a past life where she had stolen people's power. The higher guide said that repair of that karma will also be part of the pyramid of love, and that this project will incorporate Karen's life purpose of re-empowering people. Vasan went on to say, "The pyramid of love has to be an actual creation in physical form." Karen felt some trepidation about creating it properly, saying, "This type of art is my weakest skill." Her patient guide assured her that it could take any form, and that Karen simply needed to be open and willing to receive the guidance that would be provided by her many spirit helpers.

When Karen asked if creating the pyramid would completely remove the obstacles, Vasan replied that there was another issue that had to be addressed. We requested more clarity, and Karen described seeing a forest. That vision expanded into a pristine location for "sacred space" in her local area that she could use for healing. Asked if this temple space already existed, Vasan said, "No." Karen was to create a sacred space, in the proper location, which Vasan would guide her to and help her develop over time. However, before this could be done, Vasan explained that Karen needed to work with and release another layer of ancestral energy in a shamanic ceremony. "You need the power of shamanic medicine to do it," she added, "and I will help you remove all of these blocks." I asked Karen if she had the ability to follow through on this task. She replied that she did, and also had friends who could help her with the ceremony.

Next, we wanted to know if there was any additional resistance to Karen stepping fully onto her chosen life path as a healer. Vasan indicated there was more to clear on her father's side. As information on this issue unfolded, I strongly felt that we were dealing with an inherited curse. Vasan confirmed my intuition. Karen's father had suffered a stroke; her brother had been injured, and later also had a stroke; and her nephew needed extensive surgery due to a hand injury. All of this damage occurred on the left side of the body and was connected, Vasan said, to injury to the "feminine side." Karen had seen this in a plant medicine journey, and was aware of also carrying this curse as a block to the flow of her own feminine expression.

Vasan explained that part of Karen's life purpose is to clear this curse in herself and her ancestors. Following that, she would gain the ability to clear curses and perform remote healing on other people, as well. I explained in detail how curses could be energetically unwound using specific shamanic techniques. Karen was comfortable with the process, and I urged her to inquire if she could begin unwinding this inherited curse right away. Her guide said "Yes," and Karen responded that her hands had already begun to perform the procedure.

"Healing others in the imaginal realm is very potent. I will help you with this work," Vasan said. "You will feel in your body what is wrong in other people and then heal it using your own body as the surrogate for that person." Karen was to place her hands on her own body in the place where the wound was on the other person and visualize using her hands to heal the other person's wound. After a brief pause, Karen said she was now physically treating her hand as her nephew's hand, and could feel his injury being healed. The remote healing skills were all very clear to her now.

We asked if there was anything more to be done. Vasan sent Karen the quality of courage—the courage to ask for help when she needs it. She was directed to ask for support and guidance from all of her spirit guides. "And yoga," her beautiful helper added. "That is an important practice for you."

Vasan then stated that this was all the work we could do for now, and she gently conducted Karen back to the gateway. Vasan had one last reminder. "Don't forget that you are a soul in a body." They said their goodbyes and Karen returned through the arch. I then brought her back along the pathway and up the stairs. She said she was feeling amazingly good, energized, and was delighted with the answers she had received. I congratulated her on the deep work she and Vasan had accomplished in one fluid journey, and encouraged her to continue working with this powerful guide.

Chapter 15

Consciousness as Healing

REALITY IS MOLDED BY OUR thoughts and perceptions. Shamanism, mysticism, psychoanalysis and quantum mechanics all share this understanding. Thus, moving from one reality to another requires only a change in one's awareness. Our perceptions are generated by numerous factors, one of which is the state of consciousness we hold. Mystics have always taught that the basis of all reality is consciousness and that it is unbounded, infinite, eternal and unified. Hermetic wisdom teachings state: "The Universe is Mental—held in the Mind of THE ALL."[12]

Thus, Consciousness, Mind and Spirit are not singular and distinct concepts but refer to the state of being a Unified Whole, which only appears divided once we think, observe or talk about it. In other words, separation is an artifact of our own fragmentation, and this illusion of separation can give rise to numerous misunderstandings.

All health issues, no matter their source, ultimately consist of consciousness or energy in some form. Therefore, virtually any condition, dis-ease or problem can be addressed using energy healing modalities, and this is especially true in the beginning stages of illness. To be clear, I am not suggesting that one engage spirit guides to set a broken bone, perform an emergency appendectomy, or heal any other acute medical condition.

However, even acute physical ailments are connected to the greater whole in a person's life. From the perspective of Spirit, there are no accidents and no mistakes. This includes not only all illness but death as well. It is my understanding that each person's time and method of death is known and has been agreed to by that being prior to incarnating. Everything happens for a reason, but this reason may be far beyond our human comprehension. As the saying goes, we are all spiritual beings having a human experience. There are many factors at work directing our lives to fulfill our soul's intentions for the experiences we choose for each incarnation.

The case studies give examples of conditions that can be addressed by the techniques outlined in this book. The main focus of my work has been healing at the personal level, primarily addressing chronic conditions of mind, body and spirit. It is critical to address this individual healing, yet we must also face the additional layers of suffering that we all carry.

Behind, or maybe underneath, our singular disorders are the strata of our intergenerational and collective trauma. I believe these represent the next frontier in psychology and healing. Intergenerational trauma is just as it sounds—distress passed down from one's ancestors, which forms another layer within the larger collective field. The archived energy that we all share by being a member of the human species is our collective trauma, and we carry it in the transpersonal realm. In each of us is embodied a holographic replica of our collective ordeals that, like any archived energy, informs our reality, compounds over time and remains active until it is addressed and resolved.

Again, our collective trauma consists of many millennia of genocide, racism, sexism, slavery and subjugation, war, dictators, natural disasters, displacement, intergenerational trauma, and the desecration of the Divine Feminine that lives in all of us. For example, every person in the United States is steeped in the vibration of the unconscionable genocide of Native Americans and barbaric enslavement and abuse of the ancestors of African Americans. Much of this is still ongoing today.

In addition to these obvious but tragically neglected energetic reservoirs are less-evident categories of suffering. We have each been born into a society of trauma that, for the most part, is completely unrecognized because it has become normalized and even institutionalized. The immediate and unnecessary separation of a newborn from their mother, including the quick cutting of the umbilical cord, is a simple example. We don't even give this immense shock a second thought because that's just the way things are done—even when we know it is a brutal and painful experience for the infant. Why do we do this? It is an outgrowth of our own experience, our piece of the collective trauma.

As I have mentioned, our anguish does not dissipate over time, nor does it resolve by itself. It remains an active part of our consciousness and serves to create the world we experience by influencing everything we perceive from an unconscious level. Furthermore, archived trauma directs energy along neural pathways that even inform who we understand ourselves to be. Both intergenerational and collective traumas are passed down to future generations epigenetically. This has been well documented among Holocaust survivors and in other research. Trauma is also transmitted emotionally and behaviorally from parent to child, and societally through education, culture and religion. I believe a spiritual mode of transmission also exists—whether by karma or by some other energetic process.

These layers of distress are stacked upon each other and cry out to be addressed and resolved, and this must happen for humanity to evolve spiritually. Thankfully, we now see some of this collective healing playing out on the world stage, as humanity awakens to a greater realization that all suffering affects everyone: victim, perpetrator and witnesses alike. We are becoming more mature as a species and more willing to recognize the symptoms of suffering for what they are. It is encouraging to see collective trauma becoming its own field of study, addressed in cutting-edge psychology and international symposia. However, there must also be a greater awakening of spiritual awareness and enlightened consciousness to confront the massive problems we all face. I do not think we will solve these immense and complex challenges without acknowledging, accepting and engaging our spiritual nature and our basic inseparability. This is the spiritual awakening we are immersed in now.

The processes presented in this book have mainly focused on emotional and psychological healing. We can, however, expand the shamanic journey methodology to help solve other classes of problems. One example of this is a student who contacted me for insight into a legal issue. She wanted to receive input from the Akashic records to determine the moral implications of different potential actions, seeking guidance for the best path through her dilemma. Utilizing the shamanic journey and calling in a legal-expert guide, we received detailed information on all the aspects she wanted to investigate. I was surprised by the extensive knowledge and insightful advice from this spirit helper, whose vast perception was impressive. I encourage clients and students to contact appropriate guides to obtain answers to questions with which they struggle. As omnipresent spirit beings, innumerable guides are ever available and desire to help us, but we must <u>ask</u>.

The following case study chronicles a client with various conditions and highlights the ease of dealing with diverse problems in a single healing session.

* * *

Peggy called me at the urging of her friend Cynthia, who had previously done extensive work with me. When I asked the nature of her concerns, she told me she had a number of issues: macular degeneration, anxiety and depression, insomnia, mental rumination, a lack of energy, and intense envy. I replied that this was an eclectic list, and we would see what her guides had to say about each point.

Peggy arrived at my home early and was very eager to begin. She was an older woman with penetrating grey eyes and a melancholy smile. I ushered her into my healing room and gave her time to take in the energy of the altar. After giving her a brief overview, I invited her to stand next to the altar and join me in opening sacred space and calling in our spiritual support. I discussed the basics of aura cleansings, and she told me she was familiar with energy work. I then removed several layers of thick, stagnant energy from her and sent them into the ground. Peggy felt lighter and less constrained after the cleansing, and said she had enjoyed the sensation of being cleansed with my large black feather.

Following that, I seated Peggy in front of my altar and explained that she would use a stone to extract more clogging energy from inside her body. I guided her to pick up my large black tourmaline and hold it in her right hand. As I walked her through the process, I noticed she was skilled at the procedure, and she reported that a great deal of dense and sticky energy came out of her body and into the stone. I guided her to discharge it all through my altar and into the ground.

We moved on to address the entities I suspected Peggy harbored. She also proved to be adept at this process, pinpointing and expelling several interfering beings without difficulty. The final one was different. It was extremely devious and full of trickster energy, and Peggy felt strongly that this was the disrupter of her peace of mind. With my direction and the supervision of her guides, she succeeded in corralling and expelling it at last; she said it was like getting rid of an itch that she couldn't reach. I questioned her about her ability to complete the process by herself, should more entities surface over time. She assured me that she could and recorded a few notes on her phone regarding the sequence and wording.

Next, I gave Peggy a brief overview of the shamanic journey, and she elected to sit at my altar for the process. I darkened the room and, when she was comfortable and deeply relaxed, led her down the steps. Once she was through the gateway, I directed her to call for a higher guide. As she did this, a being promptly appeared to her. I asked her to describe him and, after she did, I suggested she ask him his name. He replied, "My name is Roscoe." That name struck me as odd, and I directed her to ask Roscoe if he was of the light. He replied that he wasn't sure, which instantly disqualified him as a guide. Peggy called again for a higher being, and the next one to appear was a lovely female spirit. This guide assured us she was of the light and appropriate for the journey.

I directed Peggy to ask her helping spirit to take her to the primary cause of her macular degeneration, and she was transported to a scene where she saw a dead man with a spear through his eye. Her guide confirmed that this was a past life in which she died in battle. The angel explained that this violent death had left Peggy with an energetic imprint of the trauma, which transferred to her current lifetime. This imprint was now manifesting as macular degeneration to finally be resolved. I encouraged Peggy to ask for any healing and restoration the spirit being could provide. When she did, the guide responded by putting balm into her eyes, which felt deeply revitalizing.

I suggested that Peggy ask if this past-life wound was the chief cause of her macular degeneration. The spirit helper confirmed that it was one but that there were other issues, too. We asked for assistance in healing these, and the higher guide replied that the primary problem was the intense archived anger Peggy was holding. Peggy immediately requested healing for this anger and reported that her spirit helper put clear water into both of her eyes to begin the process of releasing it.

The luminous guide then told Peggy she did not need to review the sources of the anger and instructed her to immerse herself in cold, clear water to remove the aggregate energies. I asked her to inquire whether the water needed to be physical or if it could be spiritual, and the spirit being replied that it could be spiritual water. I recommended that Peggy ask to have the clearing with spiritual water, and she reported being led "into a strong, turbulent, but clear river" into which she completely submerged herself. This living water washed away considerable debris, including her anger, and she felt powerfully cleansed and refreshed. When she emerged, the higher being confirmed that this archived anger had been discharged, and Peggy thanked her for the crucial release.

Next, we asked the spirit being to show us the cause of Peggy's anxiety and depression. Immediately, she reported seeing herself in infancy when, at about six months of age, she had contracted polio. She said she had always been aware of this; her mother had told her about it when she was a child, but she had never really thought about it. Peggy watched with growing concern as she was taken to the hospital by her parents and put in a small room all by herself. She stayed in that room—completely isolated and alone—for a week, and was only attended occasionally by the busy nurses and doctors.

Peggy saw that her parents had visited her daily during that time, but they could never stay long because they had other children at home. She reported acutely experiencing the utter abandonment she had felt during that time. "There I was," she said, "all alone, powerless to care for myself, unable to comprehend what was happening, and at the mercy of total strangers." Peggy was strongly impacted by this distressing event and keenly felt the infant's intense emotional anguish.

I asked Peggy to request her guide to enlarge the scene spiritually, allowing us to see an expanded scope of this incident. As her perception increased, she realized that she had, in fact, never been alone. Archangel Gabriel had been in the room with her the entire time, protecting and watching over her. This awareness was profoundly comforting to her and helped her to release much of the pain she carried.

I guided Peggy to pick up her infant self and to hold her close to her heart. As she did this, she assured the baby that she would always be there for her and would never abandon her. She then told me that her caresses, soothing words and compassionate feelings had instantly calmed and comforted her infant self. I recommended that she do this for herself whenever her feelings of anxiety and depression arose. Her spirit guide chimed in to say that she could be called upon at any time for protection and healing, and that she is always present.

Peggy said this experience felt enormously healing and reassuring, and she promised to remember it. After a few minutes, once the infant was calm again, Peggy replaced her in the hospital bed and said goodbye. She then conveyed to me her readiness to continue on her healing journey.

Peggy's troublesome envy—which hung over her like a thick, dark cloud—was the next issue we wanted to investigate. When we asked the higher guide about it, she informed us that the cause was Peggy's long-standing habit of thinking that everyone else was better than her. The helping spirit wisely pointed out that this was simply not true and was mostly fantasy and projection. When we asked what we could do to remedy this, the guide replied that she would work with Peggy daily to dismantle the habit. Peggy stated that she wholeheartedly agreed with this solution and was eager to begin.

I had the feeling there was a self-inflicted wound within this pattern. I perceived it as a thorn in Peggy's inner being, and when asked if this was accurate, the guide confirmed that it was. I queried Peggy to see if she wanted to remove the thorn, and she replied with an emphatic yes! I suggested she make this request, and when she did, she reported that the spirit being hesitated. We inquired about this surprising delay, and the guide replied that although she was not aware of it, Peggy thought that if the thorn was removed it would leave a big hole in her psyche.

To alleviate this worry, I told Peggy her spirit guide could repair the void and asked what she would like to place in the space once the thorn was out. When she enumerated a list of qualities she wanted, her helping spirit promptly removed the thorn and filled the hole with the desired energies. I asked Peggy how it felt, and she described it as a most magical experience. The higher being reminded her that, as the two of them continued to dismantle her habitual envy, she would fill any additional holes that appeared. Peggy was visibly relieved and cheered by this information.

At this point, we both remembered that Peggy wanted to work on her problem with insomnia. When asked about it, the guide replied that we had already taken care of that issue, explaining that the final entity—the troublemaker—that Peggy had expelled was the cause. This was a pleasant surprise and confirmed what she had felt about that devious being.

We then moved on to address Peggy's complaint about her lack of energy. She had researched this topic online and discovered that it could be related to her penchant "for keeping so much of [her] personal material suppressed." I asked her to elaborate on this, and she explained that if she used large amounts of her psychic energy to suppress her feelings, there would be none left for her life. I agreed that this was very likely the case, which her guide promptly confirmed. We asked what we could do to address this situation, and the spirit being displayed what Peggy described as her "large collection of suppressed traumas." She told me she could see each ordeal "in its own little bubble, or compartment." She asked if her guide could clear some of these, since she had accumulated and buried numerous experiences throughout her life.

Immediately, Peggy reported seeing the higher guide reach into her energy field and empty each bubble, one by one. When she finished, the helping spirit "smoothed and healed my entire energy field," Peggy said. The luminous being then informed her that these suppressed wounds served no useful function but were purely baggage that she did not need to process. Peggy said the experience of having the bubbles cleared was extraordinarily healing and left her feeling younger, lighter and more energized as a result. I told her I was pleased that her traumatic imprints were gone.

We then asked if there was any more for us to do and were informed that the journey was complete. At Peggy's request, the guide took her back to the gateway. I prompted her to thank her helping spirit, who then reminded her of the work they would be doing daily. I confirmed that Peggy was ready to return and brought her back up the steps into her everyday life.

As I watched Peggy reorient to the room, I couldn't help noticing how much her appearance had altered. She did look younger, with more color in her cheeks, and her smile was a happy one. When I commented on this, she replied that she felt revitalized and that it had been an illuminating experience. I told her I was very pleased with how her journey had unfolded and encouraged her to continue working with her radiant guide. She promised she would do the work they had agreed on and was sure she could accomplish her goals. We then thanked all of our guides and closed sacred space.

Months later, I contacted Peggy to see how she was doing. She told me her macular degeneration was still present but had not progressed at all. I asked her if she had continued to collaborate with her guide, as they had agreed. She said that she had addressed many other concerns with the spirit being but had not specifically asked for more help with her eyesight. I congratulated Peggy on her continued work with her guide and encouraged her to add dedicated focus on her macular degeneration until she fully healed it. She agreed it was a good idea to start directing more attention and effort to her vision.

* * *

Over the decades of working with clients' guides, I have found that a key to obtaining superior results is asking the right questions. In general, spirit beings will answer the question one asks, which is not necessarily what one means. The facilitator needs to focus specifically on the client's condition and speak clearly about it. Additionally, the practitioner should tune in to their strengths, abilities and gifts to become ever more adept at using and fine-tuning them to fit each client and process. Creativity, curiosity, persistence and thinking outside the box are vital aspects of this energy healing work. It is also crucial to ask the higher guides for help whenever the process gets stuck or bogged down. Spirit beings will occasionally offer suggestions and advice, but most of the time they won't unless you make a direct request.

My session with Katherine demonstrates creative thinking. She was a smartly-dressed middle-aged woman who came, decades ago, "to get rid of my anger at my mother." She consistently blamed her mother for numerous things that she felt had gone wrong with her life. Katherine had tried many types of therapy and different techniques to release her anger, but none of them had touched the real essence or source of the anger she felt.

As we went into the shamanic journey, we requested to go to the core of Katherine's anger. The higher guide took her to her early childhood, where she witnessed and cleared many issues, but her anger remained untouched. Next, I suggested she ask her helping spirit to provide insight on her experience in utero. Katherine reported finding several issues to resolve there, which her guide immediately cleared. Still, the anger persisted, and I realized the solution must lie even farther back.

I recommended that Katherine ask to travel back to before her conception to review her soul script, agreements, and planning she had engaged for this incarnation. I specifically directed her to find out why she had chosen this particular woman to be her mother. Once Katherine was there, the spirit being laid her life plan out before her, and she was astonished by what she saw. When I asked her why she had chosen her mother, she replied emphatically, "I didn't choose this woman to be my mother. I demanded that she be my mother!" With this sudden recollection, all of Katherine's entrenched anger instantly evaporated. She explained that she saw her life's plan and the purpose behind every one of her "negative life experiences" that she had blamed on her mother. It was a life-changing vision. We were both stunned that this powerful revelation entirely re-solved her lifelong anger.

For the practitioner, personal experience is priceless, and one's direct participation in energy healing work is always the best teacher. Reading this book will give you many good ideas about how to proceed, but actually doing the energy healing work will reveal how you do it. Each person I have trained to use these techniques has applied them in their own way. Everything you have ever experienced or encountered will likely be called into play, in addition to your unique therapeutic gifts, when you offer selfless service to another. There is no need to become anything other than who you are to use the information presented here to help others. It is enough simply to begin. I will also note that Spirit does not practice "dress rehearsals." Healing occurs only in the present moment, and this is how one learns.

Each of the techniques presented in this book is modular. Each ener-gy healing procedure can be combined with or used in conjunction with many other healing modalities. I, and many people I have trained, have used them in this manner with great success. Examples of these other heal-ing modalities include Reiki, bodywork, massage therapy, acupuncture, reflexology, physical therapy, psychological therapy, therapeutic touch, sound healing, hospice work, spiritual healing, plant medicine journeys, shamanic practices and more.

The practitioner can adapt the language they use to describe the various processes to fit the client's mindset. The techniques presented are driven by the direct perception and consciousness of the client. The facilitator's suggestions and encouragement keep the process flowing. Bodyworkers, therapists and even acupuncturists I have trained have told me they seamlessly interweave these techniques with their disciplines. Clients can be guided into an altered state to facilitate a particular process and then redirected back to the original therapeutic method employed. If, for example, an energy complex, block or archive is perceived in the body and does not respond to other techniques, the practitioner can incorporate any of the processes presented here that feels appropriate. Once the block resolves, the healing session may then continue smoothly.

If you encounter an insurmountable issue, the spirit guides can offer suggestions and alternatives that may not be apparent or even considered possible. Sometimes, intractable problems may be more than the client is ready to heal, or there might be compounding conditions that are beyond the scope of the guide's permitted intervention. I have found the beings of light to always be forthcoming and truthful about a client's situation when asked. The following case study illustrates a complex problem that remains unresolved.

* * *

Kelly was a returning client, an older woman who had worked with me some years previously. She called to explain that she wanted to work on preparing for her death. We chatted about her feelings around her passing, and I asked her if her death was imminent. She replied that it was not, but she thought it was always good to be ready for her death. I agreed and said we could ask the guides for more input. Kelly then mentioned that she suffered from chronic insomnia and admitted that she had been on medication to treat it for decades. She was afraid to get off this drug because she feared she would not sleep at all. She had tried stopping it, but the resulting sleep deprivation caused her to not be in her body, and to have accidents. I told her we would ask the spirit beings what we could do to help her.

I was happy to see Kelly again and admired her turquoise necklace, which set off her silver hair. We hugged, and I welcomed her into my healing room. Once she settled in, we opened sacred space and called in our spiritual support. She remained standing as I performed three energy cleansings on her aura, and reported that they made her feel more present in the room. I reminded her that she needed to enact these cleansings regularly at home.

Kelly took a seat in front of the altar, and we focused on the entities I sensed in her. She was quickly able to uncover several creatures, which she expelled and sent on their way. I inquired about her ability to carry out this process by herself in case more surfaced, and she replied that she thought she could.

I refreshed Kelly's memory of the shamanic journey, for which she opted to lie down. I guided her to relax and then led her down the steps into the realm of the unconscious. She called in a higher guide and reported being greeted by a beautiful, angelic female who, when questioned, was found to be appropriate for the journey and of the light. I directed her to ask to see the original cause of her insomnia. Instantly, Kelly saw "a jumble of wires, resembling a tangled slinky" in her brain, and the guide told her these were her neurons. The angel explained that this snarl was caused by "working too much and having too much work to do." I asked Kelly if this was true, and she confirmed that this was her current situation. I suggested she inquire how we could remedy it, and she asked, "Can you heal this mess?" The spirit being replied that it could be done but it was an intricate and laborious process.

I suggested that Kelly ask if her spirit being would call in another helper who could assist with this healing. Moments later, she reported that the angel had called in her own teacher, who quickly appeared in Kelly's vision. "They are now working together on untwisting the wires," she added. I then asked her to inquire if other factors besides overworking were involved with this brain tangle. They replied that Kelly also had a physical and psychological dependence on the sleep drug she had been using, saying it was for short-term use, but she had been taking it for many years.

Kelly and I discussed this problem, and she admitted that it was true. Her doctor had advised her to stop using it, but she had steadfastly refused. I encouraged her to ask the guides how she could end her dependency, and they advised her to wean herself from it gradually, over about six months. Kelly was more than a little afraid of relinquishing her medication and repeated her fear of getting into some kind of accident due to sleep deprivation. I suggested she ask if the spirit beings could help her with the weaning process, and they replied that they could help a little, but she would have to do her part. They explained that once Kelly was off the drug, they would then be able to heal her chronic insomnia at the energetic level. She said she would talk to her psychiatrist about tapering off it and see what he advised.

Over the years, Kelly had done a great deal of inner work on herself. She had been through many past-life experiences, she said, where she had been oppressed and felt that she had now totally liberated herself. I asked if she had faced and healed much trauma from her current lifetime. She answered, "Yes, but not as much as in my past lives." I asked if she wanted to clear any remaining present-life trauma, and she replied affirmatively.

I directed her to ask the two angelic beings to please clear as much of her archived present-life trauma as was permitted. Once they began, Kelly excitedly reported that she could distinctly feel them "cleaning out my meridians" and was surprised that she could perceive it happening in her physical body. The spirit guides explained that the process was extensive and would take a while to complete, so they would continue working on it over time.

At this point, Kelly again brought up the topic of her death and her desire to be prepared for it when the time came. We asked the angels if they could advise her on this issue, and they replied that they could not. I suggested she ask them to please send in a light being who could help, perhaps a death-preparation specialist. Kelly asked, and immediately a thin male spirit being came in, whom we queried to ensure that he was of the light.

Kelly proceeded to ask him a series of questions and reported that his answers were extremely helpful. He said he was always available to help her prepare for her life's end, and she asked him if there was something she could begin to do now. He replied cheerfully, "You're already doing it!" When I asked what this meant, Kelly disclosed that she was taking a class on exploring death at a community college. I was curious to know if the guide could tell us if Kelly would be passing in the near future, and he assured her that she would not be dying anytime soon. He added that it was always good to think about one's demise and prepare "because all incarnated beings die."

I suggested Kelly ask whether there was a preferred time for working with this specialist guide, and he replied that he would help her in her dreams, in her meditations and in waking life. She responded with delight and gratitude to know him and said she was looking forward to partnering with him for ongoing instruction.

The spirit being then advised us that we had done all we could for the day. I directed Kelly to request to return to the gateway, and she was there. She then thanked all the guides who had assisted her in her journey. When she was ready, I brought her back up the steps and gave her a few minutes to acclimate to the late-afternoon light. She was in an elevated mood and told me she felt much better about herself than before our session, and was very grateful for the healing work we had done. Kelly still wasn't sure she could get off the sleep medication, but she agreed to talk to her psychiatrist at her next appointment. We again thanked all our spirit helpers and closed sacred space.

When I followed up with Kelly months later, she admitted that she was still taking the drug and had not even attempted to wean herself from it. Even though her psychiatrist kept encouraging her to discontinue it and offered to help her through the withdrawal, she was still too afraid of the consequences that could result if she stopped. Again, I urged her to do whatever it took to end her dependency on the drug and reminded her that the guides would be able to heal her insomnia once she was off it. I suggested asking Spirit for help and encouraged her to give it an honest try. She again promised to work on her fear and resistance so that she could take this critical step toward wholeness.

* * *

As this last case study indicates, the higher guides are not always able to resolve every issue. Much of the energy healing that is accomplished depends on the person's willingness to take continued responsibility for their self-care. There are some health conditions that an individual must heal for themselves. These illnesses are generally chosen before incarnating because the soul desires to have the experience of living with them and, sometimes, healing them.

Spirit beings are always with us and know what is in our best interests, but can never act without our permission and cooperation. When restoration to good health is dependent on the client's behavioral changes, resolution can sometimes be out of reach since not everyone is willing and able to make the adjustments required to heal fully.

Chapter 16

Ghosts and Their Release

Occasionally, I've had clients who have had problems with ghosts. Some of them were aware that the issue involved a ghost, and others wanted to know why they were having bad luck, having odd things happen, or why something was going wrong with their house or property.

First of all, what do I mean by a ghost? I am defining a *ghost* to be a human who has died on the physical plane, yet—for whatever reason—is still attached to it. The ghost, who is now residing in the astral plane, believes it is still alive on Earth. Actually, it is still alive; it's just not incarnated in a physical body. Most commonly, the person died suddenly and possibly violently and ejected so quickly out of the physical body that they did not register the transition.

As Dr. Daniel Foor states in his book *Ancestral Medicine*, "Individuals who die through suicides, murder, accidents, war, or other sudden and/or violent deaths are at greater risk for having difficulty in joining the ancestors."[13] In other words, in addition to rapidly exiting the body, the deceased person has not been met by spirit guides or ancestors who could assist with the transition to the next stage of existence. This situation can result in their becoming a ghost, mistakenly thinking they are still on the earth plane, and trying to continue living here.

Other times, ghosts may be strongly attached to the physical plane out of an intense longing to stay earthbound or to remain connected to a person or a place they love. These ghosts may or may not know they are deceased, and typically they become a problem for the living only when there is a conflict of some kind. Many castles in Europe, for example, have resident ghosts who remain there peacefully for generations. The ghost may not want to leave, and the castle owner may desire the ghost to stay as a curiosity or even a tourist attraction.

* * *

Decades ago, a young woman named Tara was very attached to a ghost and came to me for help. The ghost was her friend Sam, whom she had known from high school. She told me Sam had "died suddenly in an accident, about six months ago," and that he had been with her since shortly after he died. Tara was clairvoyant; she could both see and converse with Sam. Since no one else could relate to him, Sam had formed a close bond with her and was reluctant to leave her presence. Tara had enjoyed their relationship but began to have some concerns about him sticking to her so closely. She came to see me, bringing Sam along, to find out what she should do about him going forward.

I greeted Tara and welcomed her into my home. She was wearing stylish sunglasses and her long blonde hair was in a thick braid. Since it was a hot day, I brought her a glass of water and then introduced her to my healing space. As she sat next to my altar, I asked her many questions about her relationship with Sam. She had known him well in high school and was sad he had died. As we talked, I got the impression that she kept Sam almost as a "pet ghost." She liked having him around, both as a companion and as a curiosity to impress her friends. We spent considerable time discussing the implications of this situation, and she reluctantly agreed that their relationship was probably not healthy for either of them. Once she consented to let him go, we began the process of helping him to move on.

I invited Tara to tell me all the details she knew surrounding Sam's death. She explained that he had been living temporarily with some of his high school friends in the Midwest. Tara admitted that she had not been there, but a friend who had been present relayed the story to her. One night, there had been a party at which everyone was drinking heavily. Sam was very drunk and, for some unknown reason, decided to go down into the basement to get something. As he got to the top of the stairs, he tripped and fell headfirst down the entire flight of steps onto the basement floor. He severely injured his head in the fall and died soon after. Since everyone was drunk, no one did anything until the next day, when they reported it to the police as an accident.

I stopped Tara at that point and asked her if Sam actually had tripped at the top of the stairs. She was taken aback by the question but stopped for a moment and checked in with her intuition. Suddenly, she exclaimed that Sam had not tripped but was pushed. I replied that I was getting the same impression—that his death was no accident. Naturally, Tara had a strong emotional response to this revelation and was deeply disturbed about it. We discussed the implications of this for a while, reviewing the high school friends who had been there and any possible problems they might have had with Sam until she felt ready to continue.

I then told Tara I was sure that Sam did not realize he was dead, which was likely why he remained earthbound. She asked Sam what he thought about this, and he replied that he didn't remember much about that night but didn't think he was dead. At my suggestion, we took Sam back to the night he died and walked him through what we believed had happened to him. As we did this, he was able to remember being pushed down the stairs but couldn't identify who had done it. We explained the details of what had happened—that his physical body had died of his injuries that night. He still did not remember leaving his body but finally accepted that what we were telling him was true.

As Sam and Tara thought about this situation, they understood why Sam felt drawn to Tara. He knew she could perceive and communicate with him, and the fact that no one else could see him had been extremely frustrating. As a result, Sam had gravitated to Tara and soon became very attached to her. She now understood that Sam was still "here" only because he didn't know he was dead. I advised them to consider that he needed to move on to his next life stage and that Tara might want to let him go. Since they both had been enjoying their relationship, it took many minutes for them to agree that the best thing for each of them was to part ways. I told them to let me know when they felt ready to proceed.

When they signaled their readiness, I asked Tara—who clearly had the gift of perceiving subtle energies—if she could open a portal of light. She replied affirmatively and proceeded to open one right above my altar space. She watched as a large, luminous being appeared in the ethereal portal, and I requested that she ask this guide to escort Sam on to his next assignment. She reported that Sam happily joined the being of light, and they both disappeared, closing the portal behind them. Tara stayed for quite a while to talk and process all that had happened. She knew she had done the right thing because she now felt more freedom. She said it was as if an immense responsibility had lifted off her shoulders. I told her I wholeheartedly agreed and commended her for her decision to let Sam go.

* * *

Sam was an amiable ghost who did not cause problems, but what about ghosts who create difficulty? Every case is unique, of course, and depends on the ghost as well as the circumstances. Even if the ghost is not disruptive, people who perceive the ghost tend to be uncomfortable or fearful because of folklore and other stories, societal conditioning and sensational horror films.

Things are hardly ideal for the ghost either since they are stuck in between lives and cannot move on in their progression of being. I have heard stories of ghosts becoming frustrated and even angry because they were being ignored by people around them. They did not seem to realize, even after many frustrating years, what had happened to them. The following case study details another ghost problem and how we resolved the situation.

* * *

Claudia was a forty-something Latinx who had been a shamanic studies student of mine years before. She called one early evening to ask about some specific work she wanted to do. She considered her questions to be rather odd and said she felt funny even asking me for help. I encouraged her to describe the issue, and she confided that she had been consistently unable to succeed at any of her goals. She lived on a piece of land that her parents had bought many years earlier and told me that both she and her whole family had experienced nothing but bad luck ever since they moved there. Claudia wanted to build a small house for herself on this land, but something always went wrong, and her plans continually fell through. She could not find a builder to construct her home, and there were many little problems as well. At this point, she felt sure there was an obstacle or energetic issue with the land itself, which is why she decided to call me.

I hugged Claudia when she arrived and led her back to my healing space. As she got comfortable, I admired her numerous gemstone bracelets and then gave her an overview of the process we would follow and what she needed to do to participate. We opened our sacred space together and aligned with Spirit. She immediately mentioned that this gave her a sense of peace and trust. I then proceeded with energy cleansings and observed that Claudia was highly sensitive to spiritual energies. She could feel the differences in her field as I pulled layers of shadowy energy from her aura. She commented on how much lighter she felt after these simple cleansings, so I suggested she perform them for herself regularly and gave her simple instructions to follow at home.

Next, I seated Claudia on a cushion before my altar and guided her in using my large tourmaline to pull additional thick, ominous energy from her body. She reported that she could viscerally feel this heavy energy being pulled down her arm and into the stone. I showed her how to release this residue into the ground and how to cleanse the tourmaline.

Our next step was to uncover the entities I knew Claudia was carrying. I explained what I knew about them and described what we would be doing and why. She admitted that she had worked for a woman who specialized in black magic and felt that this woman had used it on her. Claudia was very skilled in locating and communicating with several grim and malicious entities in her body and had no difficulty evicting them with the guide's help. I advised her that I strongly suspected she had more entities that remained hidden and made sure that she could complete the entity removal process by herself.

I then recommended that Claudia make a protective talisman and wear it daily. We discussed this procedure at length, and I gave her both written instructions and the ingredients to create one for herself at home. She promised she would make one the very next day and begin wearing it immediately.

Following that, I gave Claudia an overview of the shamanic journey. Once she was comfortable on her pad, I led her in deep relaxation and then down the steps into the unconscious. I asked her to call in her higher guide, and she immediately reported that a Native American man had appeared. Claudia said she was familiar with this guide and had worked with him in the past, and we determined that he was of the light and appropriate for the journey.

I directed Claudia to ask the spirit being to take her to the land she lived on and show us the root of the problems she had been having. He instantly transported her there, and she reported that another Native American man met her and blocked her way. He told her she could not enter until she made an offering to the land. She asked what kind of offering he wanted, and he requested that she leave several oranges in a specific place. Claudia promised to do this as soon as she returned home, and the man allowed her to continue.

As Claudia entered the journey landscape, she exclaimed that she could see "a dead man flying all around in a frenzy and panic." She confessed that she was afraid of him because he was dead and explained that she had always felt death in this place, which made her afraid to explore further. I gently assured her that this deceased being was there only because he was lost and confused. He was not aggressive or dangerous, just upset. I added that I thought he probably needed our help, which immediately got her attention.

Claudia asked how we could help him, and I replied that we could help him move on to a higher state of being, which would allow him to release his attachment to her land. This information calmed her fears somewhat, and I told her we needed to find out who he was and what he knew about his circumstances. Claudia agreed to do whatever was required to help him, so I directed her to ask the ghost his name. She did and reported that his name was Marvin. I then advised her to ask Marvin if he knew that he had died and was no longer in a physical body. Claudia said he did not think he was dead and wasn't sure he believed us. I told her to inform him that, to us, he was a ghost inhabiting the astral plane and not a human still living on Earth; that was the reason most people couldn't see him and wouldn't talk to him.

Marvin paused to consider this revelation and acknowledged that it would explain his frustrations with trying to ask people for help. He complained that no one answered him when he spoke; he had found this extremely distressing and reacted with panic. By this point, Marvin had stopped his frantic flying and had begun listening to us. We reiterated that he was no longer in a physical body, which meant that most people couldn't see or hear him. As he knew, Claudia could perceive him, but she was afraid of him because he was a ghost. He considered this and then conceded that he must indeed be deceased.

We asked Marvin if he would like help crossing over to wherever in the spirit realm he belonged, and he replied, "Yes, please help me." He added that he was ready to go now, so I directed Claudia to request her higher guide to open a portal and call in a spirit being who could help Marvin cross over. She reported that a radiant opening appeared, and she watched as a woman came through it. We both had the feeling that this was Marvin's wife, who was pleased to be able to collect him. We said goodbye to Marvin and wished him well as he was escorted through the glowing portal.

I told Claudia to request that the higher being immediately close the opening, which he did. I explained that it is crucial to close the portal after opening it unless you plan to continue working with it during that session. Several friends have told me about their uncomfortable experiences with open portals that had attracted numerous other ghosts in the vicinity until they closed them.

Claudia was amazed at these events and greatly relieved to be rid of the distraught ghost; she was also grateful that we could help him. She admitted that she was still a little afraid of ghosts but vowed, at the very least, to try talking to them if she encountered any in the future. This experience had been a real education, she added, and wondered why no one had ever taught her about these things before.

We then asked the spirit being if any other issues with the land needed attention, and a Native woman instantly appeared. She explained that her daughter had died and was buried there. The mother had specific requests for Claudia, which included incorporating the daughter's name into Claudia's daily prayers. Claudia asked for the daughter's name and promised to carry out the mother's wishes.

The woman also requested that Claudia create a sacred altar somewhere on the land in honor of her daughter. I asked Claudia how she felt about complying with this, and she replied that she would be happy to do it. I suggested she make a verbal pledge to the woman that she would do as she asked. In return, the woman assured her these actions would energetically free the land. We then thanked her for telling us what was needed to heal the old wounds, and she departed. Claudia expressed her great relief that we could clear these blocking vibrations so easily, and we shared a moment of quiet reflection.

At this point, the Native man who had initially confronted Claudia stated that his people's blood was also on this land, and he insisted that they be honored as well. Claudia asked him what he wanted her to do, and he gave her a list of specific requests and how to fulfill them. She assured him that she would do everything he wanted. He told her the prayer bundles she had already buried on the land were a good beginning and asked her to make three more of them. She was to incorporate the new information she had received about his ancestors into each bundle, which she promised to do.

Finally, the Native man confirmed that these actions would completely clear the energies of the land and end the bad luck that had plagued her family. We thanked him for this assurance. I asked Claudia how she felt after receiving such intense instruction, and she responded that it was an immense relief to have gained so much knowledge and insight. She thanked me for helping her find these answers.

Claudia's higher guide advised us we had done everything we needed to address the problems with the land. I prompted Claudia to thank everyone for their assistance, which she gratefully did. I then directed her to ask to be returned to the gateway, and she replied that she was there. She thanked her spirit helper again and, when she was ready to return, I brought her back up the steps into the everyday world.

Claudia was bubbling over with joy to finally understand the complicated issues that had been impeding her. She also felt deeply empowered to realize that she was capable of dealing with all of them and was eager to go home so she could start carrying out her promises. I told her that I was pleased with our success in resolving the problems and had enjoyed the intriguing session.

To conclude our work, I used floral waters, feathers and prayers to fill Claudia's aura with the energies of love, light and blessings for her long drive home. I reminded her to make her talisman and call me if she had any questions about her assignments. I also asked her to let me know how everything turned out for her and gave her another hug. She thanked me again for taking the time to work with her and resolve the problems plaguing the land. We chatted about ghosts for a while longer and finally closed our ceremonial space, thanking all our guides once more.

Claudia called several months later to give me an update on her progress. Her house was finally under construction, all was going smoothly, and there had been no further problems or bad luck. She assured me she could feel that the land was entirely cleared and at peace, and she was now very much enjoying living there. I was delighted to hear the happiness in her voice and thanked her for sharing her good news with me.

* * *

Ghost Clearing Process

Overview:

This process is for an uncomplicated removal of a "typical" ghost. It is helpful to have someone present who can perceive and communicate with the ghost to assist in the clearing process. However, one can carry out the procedure without such a person by petitioning the higher guides for assistance. My experience with ghost clearing sessions has generally been at the request of a client who could perceive and communicate with the ghost but didn't know how to resolve the situation. Sometimes I can feel the ghost, but other times I cannot, so I find it most helpful to work with someone who has a strong ability to perceive them.

None of the ghosts I have worked knew they were deceased. Frequently, ghosts refuse to believe they are dead—even after being informed of this fact—and can be rather stubborn about it. One reason for this is that the lower astral plane looks much like the earth plane, and the astral body feels like a real body to them. Therefore, they do not consider themselves to be "dead" in the way that most people would define it because they are in a living astral body in the astral plane.

As I have mentioned, a ghost may have no recollection of dying, which is especially true if the death was sudden or violent. One's demise can be quite confusing for a person unfamiliar with higher states of being, and who believes they will cease to exist after death. You may need to enter into a dialogue with them, explaining why you think they are deceased. Eventually, with enough questions and explanations, all ghosts I have encountered have finally accepted that they were no longer in a physical body and agreed to move on.

Under certain circumstances, the ghost may still be earthbound because of a strong attachment to a person or a place. In these cases, you must address the attachment issues first and resolve them. You can summon the higher guides of the deceased person to assist with this process.

There are times when a group of people may have died together: an entire family in a car accident; residents of a village overtaken by flooding; airline passengers in a plane crash; multiple victims of war or terrorism; or as a result of other incidents of accident, illness, violence or natural disasters. In such cases, it can be helpful to perform a ceremony for those who were lost. Singing, dancing, drumming, praying—or any other rituals you feel guided to carry out—can help smooth the way for their transition from the physical world.

Vast spiritual support is always at hand in these circumstances, and calling upon the higher guides or the healthy ancestors of those involved augments this support. If the land itself needs to have its energies healed or repaired to come back into balance, the spirit helpers can guide you to enact a ceremony that will help restore it to health.

This clearing work usually takes place at the actual location where the ghost has created concern. However, you can do it anywhere since the ghost can be called to you or brought to you by a spirit guide. Sometimes, a living person can journey energetically to the site to interact with the ghost. It is essential to ensure that the deceased individual successfully transitions to their next stage, which nearly always occurs via an energetic portal. I believe that an open portal also acts as a beacon to other ghosts who are stuck here. If you feel called to work with ghosts who are lost, attached or wandering, you might want to explore working with portals and higher guides in the service of these earthbound souls.

Step-by-Step Process:

1. The first step is to open sacred space with your client and call in your guides. Ideally, you want to be in the presence of the ghost and establish good communication with it.

   You can accomplish this in several different ways: visit the location where the ghost is present and summon it; ask the person to whom the ghost appears to call it into your space; create an imaginal link to the place where the ghost resides; or use the shamanic journey process to connect with the ghost or the ghost's guides.

2. Ask the ghost for its name, so you can relate to it personally and, most importantly, ask the ghost if it knows it has died on the physical plane. You might also want to get some background information from the ghost about what it knows, why it is where it is, as well as its emotional state.

3. If the ghost does not know it is no longer incarnated, explain the circumstances clearly and wait for a response.

   If the manner of death is known, it is helpful to recount the death event in as much detail as possible. If it is unknown, ask the ghost if it is aware that it doesn't need to eat, drink or sleep. Ask if people seem to be ignoring it and don't respond when it talks to them. Perhaps the ghost has noticed that it can walk through walls or perform other unusual activities. Higher guides can offer suggestions and assistance with this step.

4. Once the ghost understands and accepts its situation, ask if it would like assistance in going on to the next stage of its evolution. At this point, the being is usually ready and even eager to go on. If not, find out what is holding it here and resolve the issues, if possible. Again, you can ask the spirit guides for help with this.

5. The next step is to open a higher-dimensional portal. This is an energetic entryway between dimensions, which allows the ghost to move into a higher-frequency reality. It also permits those in that higher frequency to descend to assist the ghost in traversing the doorway.

Even if you are skilled in opening portals, you still might want to invite a higher guide to assist you. I typically call upon Archangel Michael to open the portal and help the ghost transition to its next plane of being. In some cases, it may be helpful to summon the person's deceased, healthy family members, higher guides or higher self to help with the process.

6. Once the ghost and helpers pass through the portal, make sure it is closed behind them. Archangel Michael or the guides can accomplish this if you ask.

* * *

Many years ago, I visited my Colorado colleague, Tamara, who worked as a shamanic practitioner. While I was there, Sarah, whom Tamara knew from a recent ceremony, called seeking advice concerning some property she and her husband had recently purchased. Tamara invited Sarah to come over to her cabin so she could consult with both of us. When Sarah, a tall, willowy young woman, arrived, she explained that the house was in a new development in a secluded highland valley. From the moment her family moved in, Sarah began hearing very disturbing voices inside the house. We asked her several questions about the voices and some other anomalies that she had noticed while living there.

As Sarah talked, I intuitively perceived a battle taking place on that piece of land, and I described what I was sensing. She and Tamara concurred with my intuition, and we slowly pieced together the story of a fight that had taken place between a small band of Native Americans and a group of pioneers who had just arrived in the valley. We quickly concluded that there had been many violent deaths on both sides during the conflict.

Due to the speed and ferocity of the battle, which had killed nearly everyone, they were still entrapped in their death trauma. We called out to them, explaining who we were, and described the situation as we saw it. We offered to help them cross over into their next stage of existence, to which we received some affirmative replies.

We called in our higher guides and requested they open a large portal and assist these lost souls to pass through it effortlessly and smoothly. The luminous gateway opened immediately, but no one moved to enter it, and no beings came in from the other side to meet them. Seeing this, I understood that they needed to be sung across to the spirit realm with a ceremony. I explained this to my friend, and she spontaneously began to sing "Amazing Grace." Sarah and I quickly joined in, and we were pleased to feel movement in the group of settlers as, one by one, they entered the glowing portal and disappeared into the light.

When the last pioneer was gone, we realized that "Amazing Grace" would not be appropriate or effective for the Native Americans. I quickly grabbed my drum and began singing and drumming, guided by Spirit in an impromptu ceremony. As Tamara and Sarah joined in, we all felt the Native Peoples attuning to us and our drumming and, one after another, they also moved through the brilliant doorway and into the light. We then asked for a blessing for all of the departed souls and healing for their wounds.

When the last person had disappeared, we asked our guides to close the portal and to bless and clear the land of any energetic damage that the battle had caused. We then thanked them for their service to us and the numerous deceased beings.

Sarah told us she found it hard to believe what she had just witnessed but was greatly relieved to know we had resolved the problem. We were all feeling profoundly moved and extremely grateful we had been able to help these spirit beings to move onward and that we had succeeded in clearing the land in the process.

Once Sarah had returned home, she called to tell us that all the voices and the disturbing energy were indeed gone. She said her home now felt quiet and very tranquil and thanked us again for helping her. She also felt comforted that she knew what to do if a similar situation ever arose again.

* * *

In his book *Ancestral Medicine,* Dr. Foor states: "I estimate that no more than two-thirds of the spirits of those who die in the United States make their way successfully into the larger circle of ancestors in the first year following their death."[14] This appraisal leaves a third (many hundreds of thousands!) of the deceased in the form of ghosts, most of whom become common ghosts—those who "just didn't make it across, and nobody has followed up with them."[15] Among these, Daniel states, there may also be the troubled dead, who can "pose a real risk to the health and happiness of the living."[16] I highly recommend reading Daniel's informative book if you are encountering difficult or troubled ghosts or have the desire to work with them.

Our current culture's denial and ignorance about what happens to us when we die are unhelpful at best. We all deserve to receive valid spiritual information about death and dying and how to make the transition to the next stage of life—regardless of our religious background. In the United States, we have become a death-phobic culture, which I believe represents an enormous disservice to everyone—especially to the dying, our beloved ancestors and all those who might require our enlightened assistance. Hopefully, these limited perceptions of death are transforming as humanity becomes more spiritually awake.

For any readers who are skilled in working with spirit guides and have a desire to assist those humans who are approaching their transitions, I suggest researching the topic of death doulas. This expanding field of service is of enormous benefit to the dying and their families, and could even become a rewarding career.

Chapter 17

The Eclectic Reality of Journeys

IN THIS BOOK, I HAVE presented chapters that describe the different modalities that I use, and I present case studies that illuminate real life applications of the various techniques. The reader will no doubt have observed that there are no journeys that highlight a single modality as the solution to all the issues brought forth by the clients. All guided shamanic journeys I have experienced have contained myriad problems and challenges that frequently require many, if not all, of the techniques and skills presented here. It is usually the case that each person has a variety of childhood, past life, inherited and ancestral issues to explore. Some of these can be quite convoluted and challenging to unravel.

Over my more than four decades of practicing energy healing, I have learned a tremendous amount from reading the case studies of other practitioners working in this, and similar healing fields. I am frequently impressed by the capacity of detailed case studies not only to teach me new information but to spark exciting new ideas and add creative approaches and solutions to my repertoire. In that light, I am presenting two case studies that exemplify the beautiful complexity of the journey process as well as the fluidity that is possible with a helpful spirit guide and knowledgeable practitioner. Here is the first of the two.

* * *

Helena was a new referral from a woman with whom I had recently worked. Since she lived in Europe, our communication was by phone. She was a middle-aged, professional woman with an advanced degree, who was skilled in communicating with a variety of higher beings and animal allies. Helena confided that she had chronic back pain, compressed discs and a congenital condition that had caused her to be in a cast for six months as a newborn infant. I told her that we would be able to get valuable insight on her inherited conditions and facilitate healing with the guided shamanic journey process, which I outlined for her in detail.

We began the remote session by setting sacred space and calling in all our higher guides and spiritual support. Next, Helena visualized standing under a waterfall of light as it cleansed her physical body and her energy field. I then guided her in performing a remote extraction with my black tourmaline, which had a profound impact on her. At her request, I also advised her how to perform extractions on herself using her obsidian sphere.

After the extraction, we removed several entities with the assistance of Archangel Michael. Without needing to be asked, Helena's dragon ally suddenly appeared and cauterized the wounds left by these entities as they departed. The dragon then spontaneously filled the voids that were left with a blue light of love and serenity.

Since Helena was already familiar with non-physical realms, I simply asked her to intend to go deeper to begin the shamanic journey. When I instructed her to call in one of her higher guides, an elderly woman came in. The woman's name was Ena. She was a folk healer who had been expelled from her clan and lived in a cave. Ena proved to be an ambiguous being, not purely of the light, so we thanked her and sent her away.

I suggested calling in Helena's Master Healer Guide, and Archangel Haniel instantly appeared. We asked if there were any soul fragments that we could retrieve. The first one came back in as a golden light that quickly entered her body. Then she described witnessing "a scene of a futuristic time with crystalline people." A long-lost fragment of Helena stepped forward into view, and that piece was also returned by Haniel. One more soul fragment then appeared in the form of a diamond which was installed into Helena's heart chakra.

We moved on to inquire whether Helena had any inherited damaging emotional energy that could be cleared. We were shown an archive from Helena's father and grandfather, both of whom had suffered from severe lower back pain. The source of this pain was their belief that they were obligated to figuratively "carry their families on their backs." I suggested she request that Haniel bring in the ancestor who initiated this energy program, and her grandfather promptly appeared in ethereal form. We directed Haniel to collect this archived sense of obligation and return it to her grandfather. As this was done, I encouraged Helena to inform him that he could ask to be healed from this burden. It was unclear to us if he requested this for himself, yet Helena said she felt the inherited energy being cleared from the rest of the lineage. We then asked Haniel to fill the space where this program had been with light.

An additional archive appeared that was buried in Helena's womb. Again, we requested more clarity, and Helena reported seeing the energy "as a curse, with the color red." This had originated as a genocidal curse meant to destroy family lineages which had been injected into the women of her ancestral community. It had been part of a violent war of "ethnic cleansing" against her people. I recommended that she petition Haniel to transmute this horrific inherited curse into love and light, and it was immediately cleared in the entire lineage.

We moved on to ask about any past lives we needed to address. Moments later, Helena reported that she was in Jerusalem and could see "a candle that had just gone out." This appeared to be from a lifetime where she had witnessed the crucifixion of Jesus, but had been uncertain what to believe about him. She later came to deeply believe in Jesus, and regretted that "I came to realize who he was too late." This had become an internalized feeling of guilt in this lifetime—a sense of "always being too late."

We asked Haniel what Helena needed to do to address this issue, and she replied that Helena has already made a great deal of progress. However, to complete the process, Helena must allow her faith to be complete, and learn to trust in the universe. "You are never too late, no matter how it looks," Haniel promised.

After that, Helena wondered if she had any hidden or lost psychic gifts that could be recovered. When we asked, Helena reported seeing "an alligator that was carrying something in a line of light." There was a distinctly Egyptian feel to this image, and symbols emerged representing ancient healing gifts and buried aspects of Helena's larger Self. These were reinstated into her as she requested it. Haniel told her that these would unfold over time.

Our next topic was Helena's childhood trauma, especially relating to the cast on her hips during infancy. Helena remembered that, as an infant, she felt like she "was carrying something on my back all the time." Haniel explained that this physical sensation had persisted, and eventually expanded to create Helena's entrenched belief that she carried the responsibility for everyone's burdens. This had been compounded by the inherited energy from her father that we had removed earlier, and was accompanied by a pervasive sense of guilt. "You believe you deserved this," Haniel continued. "You need to forgive yourself and let go of the guilt. I will clear the trauma template from your physical body," she told Helena, and we paused for a few moments to complete this process.

Helena then wanted to explore the emotional and psychological aspects of her tendency to carry the burdens in relationships, instead of being able to share them equally. When we requested deeper insight into this pattern, Helena confided, "I don't believe anyone else can handle the burdens. I don't think they are capable." I asked her why she carried this judgment. She sat with that for a moment, and then replied that it came from her mother. "All the women in my lineage are slaves to the family," she explained. Recognizing that she wanted to eliminate this confining belief, she asked for it to be transmuted into one of shared responsibility, equality and balance. Helena felt the instant transformation, and asked Haniel to restore the original Divine Template for her current incarnation.

Finally, we asked if there were any other issues we needed to address, and Haniel cautioned Helena that many dark beings were attracted to her light. "Place a strong intent and surround yourself with a pink light when you feel you need protection. It is important to be aware of times when you are vulnerable and to maintain this shield. And be sure to release all energies that are not yours and call back all your own energy every day." Helena reported seeing herself enveloped in gold, white and pink light, and I encouraged her to continue this important practice.

This concluded our lengthy session. Helena thanked Haniel for all the healing she had facilitated, and promised to continue the work with her and Helena's other guides. Slowly, Helena brought herself back into balanced, alert presence. I congratulated her on the deep work she had done, and observed that it would take some time to integrate all the transmuted energies. Helena thanked me for orchestrating the journey for her. She described it as "profound, very deep, and experiential," and said she felt safe and grounded in the space I was holding. "I am grateful that we came together," she added. We closed our sacred space, thanking all our spirit helpers for their support.

* * *

This next case study describes a situation in which the client is only marginally able to directly perceive what is transpiring within the journey. In this instance, the client felt that she "knew" things, without knowing how she knew, or having a clear perception of many aspects of the journey. This skill is known as claircognizance, a form of intuition that is a somewhat uncommon. Most people I have worked with are able to experience the communication with and actions of the guides as we move through different states. A large majority of this population is able to fully see— some in astounding detail—and participate in all aspects of the journeys.

For the practitioner, if the client lacks these more overt skills, the person must be guided and encouraged to identify other methods of sensing, knowing, feeling, intuiting and perceiving. I have also noticed that many clients who begin the journey process with marginal skills tend to improve steadily throughout the course of the journey, especially if their attempts are reinforced by me as being valid. I also add my experiences to enhance and encourage their awareness.

* * *

I received a text from a woman named Carmen, a young Latinx who felt surrounded by negative energies and feared that curses were somehow affecting her. I asked her if she had a good connection to her spirit guides. She replied that she is Catholic and believes in angels, but doesn't really relate to spirit guides. I suggested trying a guided shamanic journey to see if she would be able to perceive, connect to and communicate with the higher beings. She agreed to do it, since she was desperate to be rid of the detrimental energies. Since Carmen lived quite a distance away, we set up a remote phone session for the following week.

After chatting briefly, we set our sacred space, called in our spiritual support and proceeded with the energy cleansings. We then moved on to the shamanic journey. After the induction, I walked Carmen down the steps and along the pathway. She could vaguely perceive the steps and the pathway, but when we got to the gateway, she said she did not experience it at all. Remembering that she is Catholic, I asked if she could imagine a cathedral before her, and she said "Yes." She entered it, and decided to call in both the Virgin Mary and the Virgin of Guadalupe. Carmen said she "knew" they were there, although she did not perceive them directly. I replied that I was definitely feeling their presence.

We chose to continue with the journey to see what we could learn about the disturbing energies that Carmen had been experiencing. First, I instructed Carmen to ask Mary if she was the target of *daño* (intentionally sent harm), curses, or other forms of sorcery. We both got an immediate "yes" to that query. I directed Carmen to request that Mary immediately clear and transmute all of the dark energy in her body and biofield. I strongly felt this as it happened, and Carmen reported that she did feel "something shift."

Next, I guided Carmen to ask about inherited dark energy such as curses, oaths, vows or decrees affecting her and her family. She did so, and reported, "I'm getting that my mother's side is clear, but there is something dark on my father's side." Without asking for details, we employed Mary to collect this inherited darkness and return it to the ancestors to whom it belonged. We also requested that Mary advise these ancestors to ask for healing for this discordant energy. I felt an extensive cellular deposit being removed from Carmen, which I shared with her.

Both of us knew that some of this dark energy was cleared and some wasn't. To address this, we petitioned Mary to block any residual negative energies from influencing Carmen or her family. Carmen felt assured that this was done, and I told her I perceived a seal being put on the dark energies.

I then directed Carmen to inquire if any past-life issues were affecting her. Both of us got an immediate "yes." Carmen said she could sense the lingering effects of a traumatic death from a gunshot wound in a long-ago lifetime. We requested that Mary clear and heal this archived energy. I felt this as a flow of cold, clean water washing over and through my body, which I described to Carmen. Carmen said she could sense that there had been trauma but did not feel the clearing itself.

I suggested Carmen ask if she was carrying any trauma from her childhood. "Yes" was the answer we both received. It had to do with Carmen's alcoholic father, and she thought that she might have been sexually assaulted by him. She called on Mary to clear all trauma in her life resulting from her father or her step-mother. I felt this trauma energy simply evaporate, and Carmen said she could imagine it but couldn't feel it. I suggested she request that Mary replace the traumatic energies with self-love and self-compassion, which she did. Once again, although Carmen felt nothing, she said she knew this had been done.

I explained to Carmen that there might be aspects of herself that had split off due to the trauma in her past. At my suggestion, she requested that Mary locate and return any of these dissociated pieces that could be retrieved at that time. When she told me she didn't sense anything happening, I described my vivid impression of many angels bringing back numerous lost pieces and reinstating them into her body.

After a moment, Carmen reported feeling a lot of sadness. She believed she should be happy, so she found that disconcerting. I guided her to ask Mary if the source of the sadness was from Carmen's own life experiences, or if it might have been inherited. The answer we each received was that it was both of these. I suggested she request that Mary gather all the inherited sadness and give it back to the ancestor to whom it belonged, and then encourage the ancestor to ask that it be healed. Carmen stated that she knew Mary had done what she asked, even though she didn't feel it directly. I could feel the clearing very strongly, and gladly shared that with her.

Carmen then said she was feeling pressure on her neck and thought that this is where her sadness was located. We appealed to Mary to collect all of Carmen's accumulated sorrow and sadness, and transmute it into joy and love. Carmen could feel the energy in her neck shift "somewhat," and I encouraged her to inquire more deeply about the remaining sensation. After a few moments, she replied that it concerned the connection between her brain and her heart. We asked Mary to please heal and clear any obstacles, and Carmen admitted she could feel "a little of that" take place.

At this point, the journey felt complete and I directed her to ask Mary to please return her to the cathedral. Carmen said she was there, and was thanking both Mary and the Virgen of Guadalupe for their support and healing. I then guided her along the pathway, up the steps back into everyday reality. We chatted about her experience for a while longer, allowing her to integrate it more fully. Even though she had not been able to see and feel what unfolded in the journey, she did feel lighter, freer and more hopeful than before our session.

Chapter 18

Why Practice Spiritual Energy Healing?

THE ROOTS OF THESE HEALING techniques are ancient, but are they valuable to us today? In other words, does this work have a place in our modern world? The main benefit of these spiritual healing practices is their effectiveness in addressing illnesses and conditions that our conventional medicine cannot heal. I have repeatedly observed the higher guides' success in alleviating maladies for which allopathic medicine and mainstream psychiatry have little to offer. The inclusion of spiritual modalities would therefore be a beneficial, cost-effective, evidence-based addition to our health care system.

Energy healing is an exciting new frontier that will revolutionize our health care services in the years to come. As conventional medicine gradually incorporates energy healing, with our understanding of consciousness, the quantum field and the power of nonphysical realities, more and more energy healing modalities will be integrated. Mainstream awareness will again awaken to the importance of our emotional, mental and spiritual bodies and the roles they play in healing. Patients will routinely be consulted and more actively engaged in all aspects of their health care and overall well-being.

Spiritual energy healing can be made widely accessible and is well known to be devoid of harmful side effects, unlike our current system that is over-invested in both pharmaceutical and surgical modes of treatment. It can be practiced either remotely or in person since time and space do not impact these nonphysical energies. Many energy practitioners and clients can attest that healing works as well at a distance as it does face-to-face. I also believe that time is no barrier to energy healing and would love to see more research on this aspect. These techniques are adaptable and can be integrated seamlessly with many other healing modalities. Health practitioners in numerous settings can comfortably add them to their tool kits.

Another reason to employ spiritual healing techniques is their availability to all practitioners. We each possess and can focus our intention—a powerful spiritual force that we have yet to appreciate and employ in conventional healing therapies. Spiritual healing methods do not require a decade of specialized training to learn to help someone solve multiple health issues; neither is it necessary to have paranormal abilities to work with spiritual energies. What is required is an aptitude for the work, a desire to be of selfless service to others, integrity, trust in higher spiritual beings and a willingness to enter unexplored realms of consciousness.

The higher guides can accomplish an impressive scope of healing. They can inform a practitioner of various options and potential healing avenues that may be unknown or that we would consider impossible. Most health conditions are multifactorial—having physical, emotional, mental/psychological and spiritual aspects in the same presenting disorder, plus potential past-life, ancestral and collective trauma components—all of which may be relevant to the healing of the dis-ease. Tracking these myriad aspects is typically well beyond most professionals, yet simple for the guides. The use of spirit beings thus exponentially expands our capacity to facilitate healing, and these luminous guides are delighted to be of service.

After more than 25 years of teaching shamanism and leading many healing-practitioner workshops, it has become clear to me that most people can easily work with their spirit guides. An apparently infinite number of helping spirits are available to us to address any situation—we need only summon them to help us. We are continually watched over by a host of higher beings that include our guardian angels, the archangels, the Ascended Masters, our healthy ancestors and deceased loved ones, and more. This plethora of higher spirit helpers is Universal, embedded in the Divine design of consciousness and the quantum field. Along with these helping beings, there is a potentially equal number of non-helpful spirits. Thus, it is essential to be selective in enlisting light beings for healing.

For the imaginal journey work, a state of deep hypnosis is not required. The client experiences a very light trance, or altered state, that is easily attainable by most people. This enhanced awareness makes it possible for the person to communicate their experiences as they unfold. They can also ask questions or get clarification from the practitioner during the journey. The guides can take individuals deeply into material stored in the unconscious, both collective and individual. Even though challenging issues, events and memories might arise for the client, these are closely monitored by the higher beings. This allows the individual to reflect upon and assimilate much of the material as it enters their perception. Any difficult experiences are nearly always comfortably integrated by the end of the session, leaving the individual feeling fulfilled and hopeful.

The energy healing received from spirit beings happens at higher levels of consciousness and can take time to "percolate down" into the physical plane. It is, therefore, important to follow up with clients after their session to ensure that they continue to integrate their experience. Remind them to consciously embrace and reinforce their healing with daily practice and awareness and to work closely with their higher guide if they so choose. In addition, I always recommend that clients develop and maintain a daily spiritual practice of any kind since it is essential for good overall well-being.

These spiritual healing modalities connect clients to their celestial guides—an invaluable and enduring aspect of this work. Once contact has been established, most people can participate in ongoing healing and other personal endeavors by directly engaging their higher guides. In every case I have seen, the spirit helper has remained an active and recognized presence in the individual's life and has expressed the desire to continue to provide daily support to that person. This represents a vital lifelong healing resource that is provided to the client by Spirit. No one is or has ever been alone in the Universe. Everything is connected.

Engaging with higher beings is deeply rewarding and can help expand the consciousness of all those who take part in this invaluable work. Both the practitioner and the client experience opening into new awareness and potential realities beyond those they have previously known. As we explore these new realms, we can connect more palpably to the quantum field—the milieu in which we have our existence that holds infinite possibilities for our spiritual evolution. This limitless state is our very nature, and we as a species are rapidly moving toward our realization of it. It is an exciting time to be alive.

Being of service through the practice of energy healing is an enormously nourishing way to spend one's time on planet Earth while helping our fellow humans to heal and thrive. In light of the immense benefits to be gained, it is worth investigating these and other energy healing techniques further to ascertain what Spirit might accomplish on our behalf.

* * *

I hope you have enjoyed the journey through the teachings and case studies presented here as much as I have enjoyed writing about them. My intention is to give you enough of the basics to understand how these techniques work and both the motivation and empowerment to explore them for yourself. Experience is the best teacher, and your spirit guides and clients will help you. Appendix II contains letters from some of my clients for those interested in their viewpoints, realizations and perceptions of the healing experience. Most of all, may the path you choose to take through this life be one of service that brings you joy and nourishment on all levels of being.

Appendix I

Step-by-Step Processes

Opening Sacred Space

There are myriad ways to open sacred space and each practitioner will develop their unique style and routine. There is no right or wrong way as long as you come from your heart. The principle is simple: you are letting Spirit know that you are leaving ordinary life behind and entering into a space that is numinous and spirit-filled to do sacred work. Sacred space is exactly that—sacred. It is pure, safe, protected and creates an environment where all client emotions and reactions are welcome. It invites in the unlimited potential of the Divine. One is also creating the energetic container as part of sacred space. This is accomplished by calling in the beings, forces, attributes and consciousness that you wish to be present.

Before you begin, you want to completely cleanse and clear yourself and your healing space, both physically and energetically. You and the space will be holding protective energy around the entire process.

1. Ground yourself by deeply connecting your body with our planet, Mother Earth, acknowledging her presence.

2. Acknowledge Spirit in whatever way feels good to you. You may wish to open your crown chakra to connect to the celestial realms.

3. If you choose: acknowledge the 7 directions to form a sphere or bubble: south, west, north, east and center, plus the above and below (also seen as Mother Earth and Father Spirit). You might wish to call in the elements for their healing powers.

4. Call in all the spirit beings you want to attend your healing session and ask for their support and guidance. You might also want to call in ancient healing beings from your lineage—or a lineage that you feel connected to—and ask for their guidance and support. Intentionally invoking the spirit world is the key, since they already know who you are and await your invocation.

5. Activate your sacred altar, if you have one; if not, you can light incense, candles, or provide other touches that bring you joy and peace. Hopefully, you will notice a distinct shift in the energetic environment as you perform these actions.

6. Close your sacred space when your healing session is complete. Acknowledge and thank—with deep gratitude and humility—all those you invoked when you opened sacred space.

You can end by saying a closing phrase such as "So Be It," "And So It Is," "Amen," or other words of your choosing. Always close sacred space when you are finished with your healing session, unless there is a reason you want to keep it open.

* * *

Energy Cleansing Process (From Chapter 4)

1. Cleansing with smoke: with your client standing and facing you, light a dried herbal bundle* to make the first cleansing pass of the aura with smoke.

Using your intention to cleanse blocking energies from the aura and deposit them into the ground, start at the top of their head. Moving the smoking bundle back and forth horizontally in a sweeping motion, gradually work your way down the front of the body to the ground. Then have the client turn around and cleanse the back of the body/aura in the same way. If using smoke presents a problem, floral waters in a spray bottle, used in the same manner, can substitute for the herbal bundle.

2. Cleansing with feathers: with the client again facing you, use a single feather, feather fan or bird wing to sweep through their energy field.

    Again, starting at the head, use your intention as you sweep from head to toe, pushing the undesirable energy into the ground. Do this on both the front and back of your client's aura. If you don't have access to or choose not to use these tools, you can vividly imagine doing the cleansing or ask your higher guide to accomplish it for you.

3. Cleansing with light: with your client again facing you, direct them to cleanse themselves with celestial light.

    Ask them to imagine as vividly as possible that they are standing under a waterfall of celestial light. You can assist the client by describing this light and asking them to imagine the light entering their entire physical body and energy field, sweeping all discordant energies into the ground. Suggesting that the client also ask the light to cleanse them augments the process.

4. You may choose to do one or several cleansings. After completing the cleansing, move on to the next process you want to use.

*__NOTE ON HERBS:__ Both white and high desert sages have become extremely popular world-wide. As a result, they are now endangered due to the reckless and exploitive over-harvesting this limited resource. It is best to grow your own sage. If you buy it, make sure it is ethically and sustainably harvested. Other herbs also work well, such as mugwort, juniper, rosemary, calendula/marigold, lavender, bay laurel, lemon balm, hibiscus flowers or yerba santa. I have heard that palo santo is also becoming endangered in Peru. Please respect our Earth.

* * *

Stone Extraction Process (From Chapter 5)

1. Pick up the stone with your right hand and say the stone's name aloud to engage it. Remind it that you would like it to help you extract heavy, dense, obstructing energies.

2. As you take in a normal breath, intend, will, imagine, command or decree that all blocking energies come from wherever they are in your body and gather in your right shoulder.

3. As you breathe out, send these energies down your right arm and into the stone. You may feel the stone getting heavy or cold, or feel it pulling the energies out of you as you do this.

4. Continue doing this procedure, using your normal breath, until you feel the process has finished—this usually only takes a few minutes.

5. Once you have accomplished the extraction, discharge the collected energies by blowing them from the stone into the ground (if indoors, this will be the floor). Remember, it is your intention to discharge the energies that achieves this.

6. Cleanse your stone with smoke (such as sage) or waters (like rue), thank the stone for its service, and replace it on your altar using your right hand.

* * *

Entity Removal Process (From Chapter 8)

1. Once the client has identified a sensation, pain, symptom or movement, ask them to focus their attention on the place in their body where they feel it is located.

2. When they have focused their attention, tell them to say aloud to that place in their body, "What is your name?"

   The client then waits for a reply. Most commonly, they will receive a name or other response of some kind. This reply can be almost anything, so if there is one, follow it up. The names of entities appear to be arbitrary and usually not related to any human the client knows, even if it sounds like one they recognize.

   Ask the person to tell you every response they receive so you can monitor and facilitate the process. If there is no reply to that first question, simply continue with the process as described. Certain types of entities will typically hide and not answer questions, at least at first. Stay with the process, and the entity frequently will respond as you ask it more questions. If the client does not receive a name, you can address the energy as "entity" or "being."

3. Next, direct the client to say the name of the entity followed by: "You are an entity. You are not part of my body or energy field. Do you understand?"

   Usually, the entity will respond with a yes or no. Some entities know what they are, while others do not. I do not consider it worthwhile to delve into the entity's history, such as where it came from or how it entered the individual. If the entity has been with a person for a long time, possibly since childhood, it may no longer remember entering the person and might genuinely think it is the person. It is irrelevant whether the entity does or does not know what it is. Notifying it that it is an entity is what matters. If there is any doubt about it being an entity, now is the time to ask if it is a "part" of the client, or a deceased human spirit. In my experience, this is not common.

It's important to always ask the entity, "Do you understand?" This will help you get a sense of its attitude and give the client the direct experience of conversing with it. Whatever response is received, you then ask the person if they want to release this trespassing creature. If they do not, either proceed to locate other entities or end the process here. Otherwise, continue to the next step.

4. Ask the client to say aloud: "Entity, I am going to completely and permanently remove you from my body and energy field. Do you understand?"

   Again, this usually results in a yes or no response from the entity, and by asking if it understands, you will gain additional insight into its "personality." If the entity is cruel, malicious, hostile, angry or resistant, it will usually make that clear to the person by the nature of its response. It may tell the person that they will not be able to get rid of it, that they will not be able to function without it, or that something unfortunate will happen to them if they do expel it. The entity might fear that it will die or be killed if it is removed. Many entities are willing to cooperate and go along with the process, so this is to be encouraged. If the entity is hesitant to comply, the following step frequently renders the entity more cooperative.

5. The client says aloud: "We are not going to harm you. We will ensure that you are taken where you need to go next, for your own evolution. Do you understand?"

   Letting the entity know you will not harm it is a compassionate and helpful thing to do. Nearly all entities shift into a readiness to move on once they hear those words. If the person has anything they want to say to the entity before expelling it, this is the time to say it. By now, both the client and the entity should be ready to finish the process, and you can move to step 6. Note: If your client has not received any responses to the questions—particularly the last one—and neither you nor the client perceives an entity, there probably is none. You can either continue the process to detect other entities or move to another part of the session.

6. This step is the decree. Ask the client to say: "I call in the guides of this entity, and ask that you please come in and completely and permanently remove this entity from my body and energy field now!"

This is said as a command, and includes the word "now." With this decree, the guides come in, remove the entity and take it wherever it needs to go. Frequently, the person can directly perceive this evacuation as it happens. They may feel instant relief from the originating symptoms or have a sense of more internal space, peace or stillness. Sometimes the client feels as if nothing has happened, and the practitioner must discern whether or not the entity is gone. In some cases, nothing has happened, and the entity is still embedded. If you did not previously ask if this is a "part" of the person, you might want to do that now. The guides will not remove a "part" because it belongs to client's greater Self.

Occasionally, the guides either fail to remove or only partially remove the entity. Your client might report that "much" or "most" or "some" of the entity is gone. The guides who initially appear may not be able to remove the entity, in which case you need to call on another spirit helper who has more power. If an entity was not removed or only partially removed, I ask the client if they are familiar with Archangel Michael. Many people know of him, and some have worked with Archangel Michael for years. Others have no idea what an archangel is or don't believe in them. If they are unfamiliar with him, I explain that he is a very large and powerful angel with whom I work and that we will call him in to complete the removal.

7. If this step is needed, direct the client to say: "I call in Archangel Michael, and request that you please come in and completely and permanently remove this entity from my body and energy field now."

Most people can perceive the arrival of Archangel Michael at some level, and he nearly always removes the entity's remnants—or the entire entity, if necessary. On rare occasions, Archangel Michael is unable to remove the entire entity. I will then ask the client a series of questions to try to determine if they are holding on to it in any way. If they are, further explanation about entities and the problems they cause will generally help the person decide to release it. If Archangel Michael did not successfully remove it and the person is not holding on to the entity, I ask again if they want to expel it. If the answer is yes, we then proceed to an even more powerful helper.

8. Ask the client to say: "I call in Infinite Source Energy (or you can use 'the Cosmic Christ') and request that you please remove this entity completely and permanently now."

   This request has never failed unless the person is still holding on to the entity. Once it is gone, the client usually feels both a sense of relief and more spaciousness. They can then request that the higher guide fill any void created by the entity removal with light, love or other energies of their choosing.

9. Repeat the entire process as many times as necessary until no more entities are detected. It is common for clients to have more than one creature to expel. To conclude, ask your client how they are feeling now.

* * *

Guided Shamanic Journey Process (From Chapter 9)

1. Begin by giving the client an overview of the process that allows them to feel safe, relaxed and ready to proceed.

2. Use an induction technique including progressive relaxation, guided visualization, deep breathing and release of all tension, thoughts, ideas and expectations to promote a fluid entry into an altered state.

3. Once the client is very relaxed and breathing slowly, have them imagine standing at the top of a flight of 10 steps leading down into their unconscious.

4. Ask the client if they can perceive these steps. If so, begin walking them down. If not, have them imagine the steps as vividly as possible

and then start the descent. Be sure to describe each step as they reach it, counting down slowly from 10 to 1.

5. At the bottom step, tell the client they have reached the bottom of the stairs and that a path stretches out before them. Ask if they can perceive this path. If so, proceed; if not, ask them to imagine the path—as clearly as they can—extending before them.

6. Direct them to walk along the path until they reach a stone gateway (or another portal, if you prefer) and request that they let you know when they have walked through it.

   The client is now in a light trance state in a nonphysical reality and ready to start the journey. Make sure they can describe to you what they are experiencing throughout the session. This capacity to narrate experiences varies considerably with each individual, yet all can usually communicate clearly enough with proper guidance.

7. Ask the journeyer to call in a higher guide and to let you know who comes in to be with them. This normally takes less than a minute.

   Determine whether it is an appropriate helping spirit for the work you want to do, and ensure that the being is of the light, as described earlier. Frequently, the client asks me how to call in a guide. I tell them to state aloud: "I call in a higher guide." Sometimes the first being to appear is an overseer, especially if it is an archangel or a religious figure. They will tell you this if you ask, and will be able to send in an appropriate spirit being to assist with the actual process. Occasionally, a deceased ancestor comes in. Most often, this being is there for support rather than being the actual guide. They will also tell you this if you ask.

8. Once the client establishes a good connection with the guide, the practitioner directs the client's interactions with that spirit being throughout the session.

   Begin by having the individual ask the guide to take them to the source of each condition they have discussed with you. Alternatively, you could suggest that they ask their guide questions regarding soul retrieval, past lives, ancestor work or any other topic that you think could be beneficial for them to explore. The journey will unfold from there.

9. Proceed from issue to issue until the spirit being lets you know that the journey is complete. At that point, have the client request the guide return them to the gateway. The person can then thank their guide and discuss any further work that they might accomplish together.

10. When the client is ready, bring them slowly up the steps, counting from one to ten, until they are back at the top of the stairs. Then help them gently return to our everyday reality, and give them time to adjust and integrate their experiences.

* * *

Cord Removal Process (From Chapter 9)

1. Direct the client to ask their spirit helper if there is cording that can be removed. If so, have them ask the guide to bring that person into their presence (this will be in an etheric body).

2. Ask the client if they can perceive this person and the cord(s) that exist between them. Nearly everyone can perceive both; if they cannot perceive the cord(s), have the client vividly imagine them. Alternatively, the client can ask their guide to augment their perception to enhance the experience, or ask the guide to remove and transmute the cord(s).

3. Direct the client to first remove the cord(s) from their own body, with loving-kindness for the learning they received from the cording. Cords frequently have many little rootlets or tendrils in the body. If this is the case, instruct the client to carefully remove each one of these tendrils. We do this with loving-kindness to avoid generating karma.

4. Once the client's side of the cording is detached, direct them to ask the other person if they would like the cord(s) removed from their body.

If the reply is no, I suggest having the client request that their guide explain to the person why it would benefit them to have the cord removed. This usually results in the person then saying yes. If the answer is yes, the client removes the cording from the other person, with loving-kindness, in the same manner as before.

5. Once the cord is completely removed from both parties, ask the client to coil it like a rope. Have them visualize a burning bowl nearby, and instruct them to place the cord into the burning bowl.

6. Direct the client to call in the violet flame of transmutation, which consumes the cord and transmutes it into light.

    Most clients report seeing the flame, but if not, ask them to imagine it vividly. They can also use this light to cleanse and heal any wounds that remain from the cording if they choose. If the client wishes to speak to the other person for any reason, let them know that this is their opportunity to do it. Then, you can allow the other person speak, if they so choose.

7. When finished, the client asks the guide to take the other person back to where they belong.

8. Direct your client to ask if there are more people with whom they have cording to remove. If there are, proceed in the same manner with each new person until the guide indicates the entire process is complete. The practitioner then moves the client along to the next healing topic.

* * *

Soul Retrieval Process (From Chapter 10)

1. Once the client is in the unconscious and connected with a light-filled spirit helper, begin by having them ask the guide if there are any lost fragments or missing pieces to be retrieved. If the answer is yes, the client asks to meet the first piece. Tell the person to let you know what they perceive and experience. If the answer is no, proceed on to another facet of the guided shamanic journey.

2. When the fragment is present, either the client or the guide will engage with the piece to ensure that it is ready to return. If it is, the client or the spirit being can collect the fragment and reinstate it into the body. I suggest bringing it back in through either the heart chakra or the solar plexus. If it does not want to return, that issue must be addressed and resolved before proceeding.
3. Ask the client to tell you when the reincorporation is complete, and then ask if there are more pieces to recover.
4. If there are, continue in the same manner until the guide says the retrieval process is finished.

   It is common for people to have multiple fragments. You can also have the client ask the soul piece or their guide if there are any specific actions or activities they might bring into their life to help each soul piece re-incorporate. Once there are no remaining pieces to retrieve at present, proceed to another stage of the journey process.

* * *

Ghost Clearing Process (From Chapter 16)

1. The first step is to open sacred space with your client and call in your guides. Ideally, you want to be in the presence of the ghost and establish good communication with it.

   You can accomplish this in several different ways: visit the location where the ghost is present and summon it; ask the person to whom the ghost appears to call it into your space; create an imaginal link to the place where the ghost resides; or use the shamanic journey process to connect with the ghost or the ghost's guides.

2. Ask the ghost for its name, so you can relate to it personally and, most importantly, ask the ghost if it knows it has died on the physical plane. You might also want to get some background information from the ghost about what it knows, why it is where it is, as well as its emotional state.

3. If the ghost does not know it is no longer incarnated, explain the circumstances clearly and wait for a response.

    If the manner of death is known, it is helpful to recount the death event in as much detail as possible. If it is unknown, ask the ghost if it is aware that it doesn't need to eat, drink or sleep. Ask if people seem to be ignoring it and don't respond when it talks to them. Perhaps the ghost has noticed that it can walk through walls or perform other unusual activities. Higher guides can offer suggestions and assistance with this step.

4. Once the ghost understands and accepts its situation, ask if it would like assistance in going on to the next stage of its evolution. At this point, the being is usually ready and even eager to go on. If not, find out what is holding it here and resolve the issues, if possible. Again, you can ask the spirit guides for help with this.

5. The next step is to open a higher-dimensional portal. This is an energetic entryway between dimensions, which allows the ghost to move into a higher-frequency reality. It also permits those in that higher frequency to descend to assist the ghost in traversing the doorway.

    Even if you are skilled in opening portals, you still might want to invite a higher guide to assist you. I typically call upon Archangel Michael to open the portal and help the ghost transition to its next plane of being. In some cases, it may be helpful to summon the person's deceased, healthy family members, higher guides or higher self to help with the process.

6. Once the ghost and helpers pass through the portal, make sure it is closed behind them. Archangel Michael or the guides can accomplish this if you ask.

Appendix II

Letters from Clients

THE FOLLOWING ARE LETTERS, SOME of which describe in detail selected experiences during the shamanic hypnosis journeys and others that are more general, talking about the benefits clients have received through the healing sessions. The purpose of including them here is to give the reader a sense of how my clients have perceived the various modalities and the impacts they have had on them. The letters also underscore some of the therapeutic messages I have tried to communicate by writing this book.

* * *

"I do not consider myself a big believer in things like soul retrieval, messages from the beyond, etc. At the same time, I think that there are a lot of unconventional healing modalities that can be beneficial, even the placebo effect. After years, decades really, of conventional talk therapy (which was mostly helpful), I decided to try working with you to clear out some residual issues.

What I like about working with you is your absolute acceptance of my experience. There is no right or wrong, no good or bad. With a traditional talk therapist, there are some things I would just never bring up, they seemed unbelievable, maybe a bit crazy. I did not feel that inhibition with you. By gently leading me through a confusing past experience and even the fog of a body memory, you helped me give voice to what I have never been able to say out loud.

Another aspect of our work together that I found helpful was the sense that we were doing something to clear out the residue, the negative energies. I might have felt foolish going through some of the clearing exercises with someone else, but with you as my guide, I felt safe and supported, able to open myself up to another path of healing."

JEAN ZAGRODNIK, SAN DIEGO, CA

* * *

"My healing session with you was quite transformational. At the time, it felt very subtle—the compassionate removal of blocks/entities that I was not even aware of—with the aid of the angelic realm. The removal of ageless anxieties allowed me, over the next few months—with renewed confidence—to ask the spirit world to accompany me in a long-overdue grieving process.

Over the past twenty years, I have become acquainted with energy healing work, specifically Reiki and had learned a heart meditation technique. I have always intuitively felt protected and guided, but when specifically asking for a guide to step forward—be present—none ever came. It was hard to build confidence in spiritual connections and left me feeling alone—in that sense.

Under your patient guidance, I eventually called upon Jesus, and he was immediately there. I had forgotten that he had been my "strength" through most of the first thirty years of my life. At thirty, I had a life experience that was soul damaging and left me feeling unworthy of his company or compassion. It was me that kept my guides from being present.

Since my healing session with you, Judy, I feel less spiritually alone, have set up an altar, and meditate on a regular basis. You also sent me off with the knowledge, confidence and tools to self-clear negative energy with the help of the telluric and angelic realms. I am beginning to reclaim some of the positive aspects of who I was so many years ago. I am thankful to you for your healing work."

MARY, MICHIGAN

* * *

"I feel that your healing work is powerful, important, and timely; cross-cultural for modern times, rooted in ancient traditions and universal in approach. I appreciate that you empower by getting rid of the middle-man between people and their guides. The Shaman is no longer the doer but someone who teaches about the many dimensions of "reality" and how to do your own work in these dimensions.

Judy, you taught me how to contact and use my spirit guides safely and effectively, as well as work with my ancestors to shift deep-seated patterns in myself and my family. You helped me better understand and navigate the Multiverse; I'm less prone to getting stuck in consensus reality and see that I am co-creator of my life.

Working on a personal, community, and global level makes it a powerful form of activism that I am now empowered to undertake. I don't feel helpless against the tsunami of atrocities facing humanity when I have this perspective.

Regular Cleansings, Extractions and Entity Removals have been invaluable during this time of upheaval, keeping me from accumulating unwanted energies and staying centered in my own knowing. Especially important during this pandemic in 2020; boundaries and immunity are the same thing! The work we did helps me stay sane during insane times. What a gift!"

JADE CHUN, LMT/JIN SHIN JYUTSU AND SPIRITBODYWORK, UTAH

* * *

"For about four years, I had an intense experience of ancestral healing. This process manifested with multiple rare illnesses, chronic pain, emotional instability and spiritual turmoil.

Working with you gave me the ground to stand upon in a very tumultuous time. Your approach worked on several different levels, but primarily it was grounded in simple spiritual truths.

Through visioning with you, I was able to get vital information about the root cause of some of the difficulties mentioned above resulting from ancestral issues. Most of the information had to do with my family and ancestral healing; murky waters to navigate.

In the sessions that I did with you at different times over about 3 or 4 years, I was able to get more keys to unlock doors that had been shut. Collectively, I was able to have a cohesive story about my family.

I am grateful to you for this grounded guidance on my journey, as I experienced many highly unusual and unorthodox things. If I didn't have that guidance, I might have gotten lost or stuck or lured by a manipulative spiritual force.

You swim in some unusual water yourself, but you always remained grounded, matter-of-fact, and connected to uncomplicated truth. This helped me trust that you are authentic in your service and not in service to some grand Ego."

MARISOL, SEBASTOPOL, CA

* * *

"I have now been using your techniques for the past year and a half and can't remember how I worked with clients before I learned them. I incorporate something with clients every week, sometimes daily. Your methods for releasing negative cords of attachment and calling in guides for assistance with soul retrieval and release of toxic energies has been an invaluable experience. I regularly use these techniques both on myself and with clients and have excellent results. I very much appreciate your experienced, grounded, organized, compassionate and clear communication and the fact that you are always available to answer my questions. Thank you, Judy!"

Victoria, MD; Colorado

* * *

(Contains graphic description of past-life events.)

"There are many times you are called to step outside of your comfort zone, the security of thinking you know what is safe and venture into a place of not knowing exactly what will happen next. I have tried to live by the adage 'Expect nothing and be prepared for anything' because even if you think your comfort zone is safe and secure you will be very surprised someday as nothing is static in this world.

I chose to visit you due to a deep restlessness about what was unfolding in my career and feeling unsure about how to proceed. Something within me said, 'Now is the time to explore deeper areas of your life and the causes of your discomfort.' The confession of being plagued by anxiety, low-level depression, and low self-worth most of my life would surprise many people as through the years the external 'me' appeared calm, capable, strong, and very, very grounded.

While there was much profound change that happened in my work with you, there are two experiences that created deep and long-lasting shifts within me. During one of the shamanic hypnosis journeys, I was met by an older male being dressed in a long robe with a hood. I could not see his face. When I asked his name, he replied, 'Melchizedek.' He took my hand and pointed to a 'fold in time.' I saw myself as a small child being used for everyone's pleasure—the scene was unclear, so we went to another time period. It was the Renaissance. There was a large, gluttonous crowd with much feasting in a large hall, almost like a small club. I was a young girl under age ten owned by someone there who brought me to these places for the sexual entertainment of the group. I was on the table dancing, exposing myself and performing acts. I had no control over what I was told to do. When I reached puberty, I was cast out and thrown into the street. Being very sick, I died there. This pedophile lifetime and others are directly related to past and current expressions/actions in society now.

I saw Melchizedek lift up the child with his right hand. The child lay in the palm of his hand and was lifted up through layers of a white, filmy substance. As this movement happened, the fractured light body of the child began coming together—retrieving sharp fragments, one by one, until complete. He then laid the child on a cloud-like substance, and other Light Beings came and tended the child as the healing continued. I was aware that I had been doing the same motion with my right hand while Melchizedek is doing this work.

I was told that I will see and know when individuals are fractured in this way. They may or may not come to a healing practice. I will pass them in the city in large crowds. I was then gifted a large crystalline sphere that I held in my right hand that will call forth all the shattered soul pieces for those individuals. I was then thanked for my courage to take this on. I was told I need to remember I cannot do all of this, only my part because the global humanity piece is so large.

Melchizedek was present again toward the end of my time in the session, when he gifted me with a significant download of energy, an initiation, which was completely unexpected and that I now carry in order to do my 'assigned' work in this world.

With experiences of this magnitude, one can feel a major energetic shift occur within the 'internal' non-physical structure of your being. Suddenly the person you identified with being seems to have slipped away and someone new is standing in the space once occupied by that person. While this can be very unsettling at first, I was given the gift of seeing more of who I truly am on this planet, the eternal being without the limitations imposed by the human body. I have learned that this shift also unfolds over time and needs nurturing to be maintained in balance since we do live on the earthly plane at this time.

I have noticed changes in my perception of situations. I am able to find the 'higher' or balancing point between two opposites. The perception more often from a place of non-judgment and allows me to see where the common ground actually exists even if it cannot be seen easily by others. I also have developed a keener sense of connectivity with others, knowing when events may occur or friends are getting ready to contact me…a definite increase in the daily use of intuition without realizing that this is what is occurring. From a deeper, more subtle level, my purpose for living this life is becoming clearer and I can more easily keep my heart open and breathe when faced with challenges on this journey.

As I say…'Expect nothing, be prepared for anything.' And always anchor gratitude in your journey. I bow in deep gratitude to you for your facilitation of this work with me…it was and continues to be life changing."

REBECCA, OHIO

* * *

I will be forever grateful to have experienced my healing session with you. Using these methods has been pivotal along my healing path and shamanic service. The experience and healing from it were profound. When I heard you would be teaching these methods, I was excited but couldn't see myself able to learn and implement them, even though you said it can be done, and by anyone. When I attended your workshop, I was very impressed by the practical work we did as students who had never done this sort of work before. This really excited me about these methods.

For me, these methods provide a more directed intentional process and interaction with the guides, healing sources, and entities encountered. I perceive the methods allow for going straight to the core of things needing work, and assisting with tackling it step-by-step, and knowing where one is in the process. My healing experience with you demonstrated to me how one can get there with precision, clarity, and deliver powerful targeted healing.

As someone who had not provided healing work to others in this way, the workshop afforded direct experience with healing resources and guidance that I have not had available to me. This was a revelation for me and gave me assurance I could move forward with these methods when needed and ready.

I am grateful to you and your inspiration to bring forth these methods for self-healing and the healing of others.

CRAIG, WASHINGTON

* * *

"I am writing to share how I have benefitted from working with you. I wasn't looking for physical healing of a disease but a rediscovery of connection to myself. I have been a life-long self-development junkie and had recently had a psychic experience involving my departed grandmother. I wanted to delve into that part of myself.

Through working with you I was able to be more embodied and could thus connect more easily to my intuition. I have learned to recognize and develop a relationship with the clear knowing that I used to dismiss when it came to me. I am still learning, growing and practicing, but now I feel like I have a map.

I feel that a large part of my healing came from a tremendous release of grief. I wasn't even aware that the ocean of tears was inside me. It was an unseen wall between me and my authentic, intuitive, connected self and you helped me dissolve it.

I am forever grateful to you Judy, for providing the beautiful and safe container, your wisdom and your welcoming heart."

RACHELLE, ESCONDIDO, CA

* * *

"We think we know. We buy into the stories told to us by our family and the greater culture. The stories tell us where we came from, and culture provides a context for how life may unfold. But for most of us in this culture, we don't know, really know, who we are because we have little connection to the spiritual energies that propel us into taking form in this life.

As a child growing up in a Christian household, I learned about and integrated stories from Christian mythology. One particular mythological character I felt a strong connection with was the Angel Gabriel. Through my shamanic journeywork with you, I have come to understand that the 'Christian' angels are spiritual energies serving mankind long before their 'adoption' into the Judeo-Christian tradition. This angel has been a guide and protector for me throughout this life and a source of wisdom and comfort.

For me, it is the shamans who opened the door to the deeper knowing of these energies. You have been pivotal in helping me uncover the spiritual layers of personal struggles that years of therapy could not reach. With your guidance in energy work, shamanic journeying and entity extraction work, I have gained insight into trauma in past lives, as well as access to the spiritual guides and protectors who have been with me all along. This process has been so useful in finding healing for the traumas of this current life."

JANE, EAST BAY AREA, CA

* * *

"I am abundantly grateful that at just the right time in my life, I crossed paths with you and that you have become my trusted teacher. When we first met, I was at a point in life where I was ready to shift my reality, my stories and to break through old and unhealthy patterns—but knew that I needed help to do so. I was fortunately referred to you, and you taught me techniques to help myself and others while also creating a clear and safe space for me to learn and grow.

You offered me tools, techniques and counsel that helped me take a deeper dive into myself to heal wounds of the past and create new pathways for my future. Through individual sessions and group workshops over the years, you have taught me processes like energy clearing and thought form clearing for myself or to facilitate with others. You taught me how to better clarify and align with healing intentions, how to create sacred spaces and altars and to remember the imperative of asking for help and guidance.

You also taught me how to work with animal allies and an unseen network of support through shamanic hypnosis, how to do home and space clearings, and the importance of taking personal responsibility for my energy and my healing path.

When I first met you, I had no idea what an amazing, long-lasting gift your presence in my life would be. Now, many years later, I can say with confidence that my work with you and the learning that I gained set me on a path to reconstruct a more self-loving, whole and aligned version of myself who is also now equipped with more tools to self-heal and re-member when I veer off of my path.

My experience of you is an embodiment of unconditional love, and it is difficult to self-judge when in the presence of such a non-judgmental guide. You have always been clear, articulate and compassionately honest in your observation and experience with me. You are a walking ceremony of gratitude who is generously willing to share as many tools and practices as one is ready to receive—whether one is looking for self-healing or to expand the offerings I want to share with my clients.

I remember our first session together...I was disagreeing with my intellect out loud in your presence about my experiences during some facilitated journey work. It seemed so 'strange' to me at that time to discover how much guidance is available and has always been available to me during my life. You affirmed my process and experience with love and support, encouraging me to dive deeper.

You are someone who has always told me that you are not here to heal me but rather to support my process to heal myself and remember my innate abilities. My work with you and your healing approach are gifts that keep giving and continue to change my life."

TRACIE TROXLER, NONPROFIT DIRECTOR, FLORIDA

* * *

"My work with you, over many years, has been among the most profound healing work of my life. I experienced a lot of early childhood trauma and had ways of coping that no longer were working for me. I had sought healing from an early age and have sought to be a help to others as I healed myself. Before I met you, I had to do a lot of this work on my own and it was easy to get into tangents that were off course. Having you as a healer and mentor has kept me on a grounded path.

I came with learning in mind, and you always had an encouraging and solid way of answering my questions. You are incredibly trustworthy. Being vulnerable to others' opinions of me, it had been hard to open up about what was really bothering me, but I always felt safe working with you.

You allowed me to take my time and get to the heart of my troubles. You helped me see that what worries and projections I carried that clouded my clarity were imaginary or wishful thinking. You offered a way to view the richness of the reality of the many realms that humans can inhabit and I was willing to leave those fantasies behind. You taught me how to discern what is true.

I will always be grateful that you helped me remember the love and gratitude I had for my mother before she died, which made our last years together sweeter. And I'm grateful that you showed me a way to be a healing presence for my father and step-father, and other ancestors who have already passed to other realms.

I always felt I was held in reverence and respect by you, just as you respect all beings in nature. You never tried to put yourself above others, though it is obvious when I work with you that you are a master, a highly-skilled, devoted and trained healer and teacher. Judy, I admire your unfailing integrity and I am proud to call you my mentor, healer and friend."

SYDNEY WALKER, L. Ac., BAY AREA, CA

Endnotes

[1] Jude Currivan, *The Cosmic Hologram: In-formation at the Center of Creation* (Rochester, VT: Inner Traditions, 2017), 8.

[2] Arthur C. Clarke, "Clarke's Third Law on UFO's", Science 159 (3812), 1968, 255.

[3] Sherana H. Frances, *Drawing It Out: Befriending the Unconscious* (Sarasota, FL: Multidisciplinary Association for Psychedelic Studies, 2001), 19.

[4] Max Planck, *Das Wesen der Materie* [The Nature of Matter], speech at Florence, Italy (1944) (from Archiv zur Geschichte der Max-Planck-Gesellschaft, Abt. Va, Rep. 11 Planck, Nr. 1797)

[5] Max Planck, The Observer (25 January 1931), https://beliefinstitute.com/quote/max-planck-mind-source

[6] Daniel Foor, *Ancestral Medicine: Rituals for Personal and Family Healing* (Rochester, VT: Bear & Company, 2017), 4.

[7] Ibid, 6.

[8] Sandra Ingerman, Awaken: https://awaken.com/2019/08/soul-retrieval-2/

[9] Sandra Ingerman, *Soul Retrieval: Mending the Fragmented Self* (San Francisco, CA: Harper, 2006), 17.

[10] Ibid, 20.

[11] Stan Grof, *When the Impossible Happens: Adventures in Non-Ordinary Realities* (Boulder, CO: Sounds True Inc., 2006), 165.

[12] Three Initiates, The Kybalion (Chicago, IL: The Yogi Publication Society, 1940), 65.

[13] Daniel Foor, *Ancestral Medicine: Rituals for Personal and Family Healing* (Rochester, VT: Bear & Company, 2017), 13 (footnote).

[14] Ibid, 163.

[15] Ibid, 163.

[16] Ibid, 163.